SHOOTING PAINS

MAIRI CHONG

IBSN: 978-1-913463-04-5 (print edition)

IBSN: 978-1-913463-05-2 (ebook edition)

For W - as always

1

'Anyone would think you wanted me dead!' Fiona spat.

Gregory paused mid-bite of his bacon sandwich. The glutenous bread soaked in oil was claggy and he had to force it over his gullet. He took a moment, knowing full well that she was waiting for a reply, or at least, a reaction. But instead, he continued to chew, glancing down at the newspaper on the kitchen table as he took another bite.

'Well?' his wife asked, apparently determined to goad him into a response.

Gregory continued to chew. The bacon was cheap, no meat to it. All gristle and fat.

'Nothing to say?' she persisted, with her hands on her hips.

Gregory looked up once more as if considering. He hated it when she stood like that. It made her look like some old fish-wife, which was absurd since she was barely in her twenties. He smiled slightly, as if at some unsaid joke. Perhaps the whole thing had been a mistake after all. A pity, he thought sadly to himself, and it had begun with such promise. He had fallen for her hard and they had married – probably in haste – but she had changed. Changed from carefree and simple, to something quite monstrous. His family had been right all along. 'Never marry a townie,' his mother had warned. True enough, Fiona had not settled into country life and things had only become worse when she had started that new job.

'I'm not letting my guard down, now that it's occurred to me,' she continued.

Gregory knew that she was half-teasing, but he didn't have the energy to continue. Having finished his breakfast, he slid his chair back, grunting as he got up.

'I'm thinking of asking Rosemary and David for dinner ...' she began, reaching out to take his plate.

Gregory was at the door. Of all the things she could have said, this was the one that might provoke a response. He turned to her.

'Don't expect me to be here,' he said.

Fiona tutted. 'Of course I expect you here. What a preposterous thing to say.'

Preposterous? Gregory thought to himself and shook his head in disgust. Since when did she start talking like that?

'You're not the only man capable of calving, Gregory. God knows why you think it. Adam has half a dozen equally capable farmhands hanging around the place. Ridiculous, that you think no-one can manage without you for one bloody evening.'

'*I'm* the cattleman,' he growled.

'Farmhand, cattleman, who cares?' Fiona waved her hand in dismissal. 'It's not difficult. You're hardly irreplaceable, no matter what you seem to think.'

She knew she'd won. She'd managed to rile him. He looked dispassionately at her and, at that moment, he did wish his wife dead. He pictured her in agony, dying on the floor in front of him.

She was pleased with herself; he could tell. He watched her smugly tip the remains of his breakfast in the bin beneath the sink. It wouldn't be so hard, Gregory thought as he turned from her. He dealt with it every day on the farm. After all, where there was livestock, there was deadstock.

Rosemary Holden leaned forward. Her dark eyes widened and her lips twitched. 'Poisoned?' she asked. 'But I don't understand. Why would you say that?'

Her friend, who sat opposite on the train, glanced sideways and smirked, probably realising only too well, that an elderly woman across the aisle might be listening.

Rosemary leaned in further. 'Well?' she hissed. 'What's he done now?'

Since she had met Fiona, the younger woman had been only too eager to regale her with tales of marital disharmony. It had been a bit of a joke between them as Rosemary herself had been going through some issues at home also. Usually, the discussions ended with the two women consoling one another. Men really were thoughtless beasts when all was said and done. Up until that day, Rosemary, who enjoyed reading up on psychology, had thought it a natural enough conversation-filler. A comradery through which all women took comfort.

'I know,' Fiona said, her cheeks glowing. 'Slowly poisoned, and by my own husband! I've not even told my sister yet. Maybe I'm overreacting, but these past few weeks, I've wondered. He was unspeakably mean when he saw me and Kenneth having a word. You should have seen his face! Like thunder it was. And he sulked for a full two days after. You'd have thought he'd caught us in the act! All we were doing was having a chat on the doorstep.'

'Kenneth?' Rosemary asked, now confused. The name had been mentioned before but she couldn't think in what context.

'Kenny. The gamey. He was seeing to the pheasants when he passed the door,' Fiona explained. 'Nice guy.'

Rosemary smiled thinly. No doubt Kenny was a nice guy. He was more than likely easy on the eye also and just the sort of person Fiona might well attract for the sole purpose of provoking a reaction in her husband. How this added up to her friend suspecting him of trying to kill her though was still unclear. But Fiona was talking once more.

'I've already told you about my skin ...' she said.

Rosemary nodded, recalling the monologue.

'Well, that's not all. It's my hair too!' Fiona pressed her immaculate brunette waves flat, and tipping her head forward, she accentuated the natural parting.

Rosemary snorted. 'If it's just greys, I'm getting them too, and that's nothing to do with my David putting cyanide in the wine.'

The elderly woman across the aisle coughed. It was a dry, little bark. She shifted in her seat once more. Rosemary rolled her eyes.

'Not greys!' Fiona said indignantly, ignoring the elderly eavesdropper. 'It's coming out. Look! My hairbrush was full of it this morning. I saw it done on a crime thing a few weeks back. He was watching it with me too. That's probably what gave him the idea. We've had mice. It might be the stuff he puts down for them.'

Rosemary, feeling rather cheated if this was all the evidence her friend had to go on, sighed. 'The hair and the skin could be a

thousand and one different things,' she said. 'They say pregnancy makes your hair fall out. Come to think of it, can't it make
you blotchy and itchy too?'

'I'm not pregnant,' Fiona said with finality.

Rosemary shrugged. 'Is that all then?'

'His manner too, Rosemary, it's been so odd. Really quite
unnerving at times.'

Rosemary arched a carefully plucked eyebrow but didn't
speak.

'You know how thoughtless he's been these past few
months?' her friend asked. 'Remember the row over Mum's
birthday? Then there was that nonsense over me taking on this
job in the first place. He's been inattentive and sulky, to say the
least. Oh, I know his pride's been dented, what with me earning
more now, but I told him that it all goes into the same pot. What
does it matter anyway?'

Rosemary nodded.

'It's not as if I've been insensitive. I told him that I knew what
he was when I married him, but he does himself no favours at
all. You know how long we've been in that rented place. I spoke
to him the other night about it. Suggested we looked out for
something of our own, off that bloody farm estate. I'm sick of
mud. Nearly blew up at me when I said that.'

Rosemary didn't speak, but inwardly she thought it unquestionably thoughtless of her friend to suggest that they move,
given that she had heard that the cottage had been a long fought
for perk of Gregory's job.

'So why have things escalated to the point that you think he's
poisoning you? Have you had another row?'

Fiona shook her head. 'Quite the opposite,' she smirked. 'He
offered to make my tea last night!'

Rosemary exhaled. 'You are joking, Fiona?'

'No, hear me out,' the other woman said. 'Let's put this into perspective. Why the sudden change, if it's not to put me off guard? He's been an inconsiderate animal for near enough six months straight. Ever since I started working for Greysons he's been insecure and narky. I'm sure he's only notched up his interest in the stupid metal-detecting to spite me because he knows it irks.'

Rosemary looked out of the window as Fiona continued to speak. Undoubtedly, work would be taxing today. Mr Greyson had already asked her to stay late several times over the last few weeks to ensure things were up to date. He didn't need to ask of course; she would have done it anyway. She was as committed to the smooth running of things as anyone. Mr Greyson knew this. She looked across at her young friend as she continued to chatter, and smiled.

It was all very well to natter about frivolities to Fiona on the train heading to the office, but when they arrived, it was quite different. Both women knew that Rosemary's role as a personal assistant to the managing director came with far greater responsibility than Fiona's as office girl. At work, they rarely spoke at all.

The train began to slow. Unsure which stop they were now coming to, she looked out for a landmark. The fields flicked by and then an industrial estate that she recognised came into view. The embankment rose steeply as she knew it must, barring further view, and the sky was obliterated as the train entered a tunnel. The neon lighting in the carriage flickered slightly. They were minutes away from Forkieth.

Rosemary began to gather her things. 'We're nearly there.'

Fiona didn't move. 'Don't you think it odd?' she asked again. 'To go from being so hostile and uncaring to suddenly changing? I'm sure that my meal last night had a bitter taste to it. I said that to him this morning. He's sprinkled something on top without my notice, probably.'

'Have you considered that he might be trying to make an effort?' Rosemary asked as she slipped her arms into her jacket.

'Why now? And what about the rash and the hair too? No, there's something not right.'

Rosemary took her gloves from her handbag and began to put them on.

'Well,' Fiona said, unable to hide the huffiness. 'If I don't turn up for work one of these days, you'll know what's happened, and then you'll feel guilty.'

Rosemary snorted.

The two women locked eyes and giggled.

The train slowed considerably and Rosemary stood in the aisle. She slipped her handbag over her wrist. The train swung and jolted slightly, causing her to clutch onto the table. She met the gaze of the elderly woman who had all this time been sitting close beside them. The woman blinked slowly and then spoke with a quiet assertion. 'Take care.'

Rosemary smiled and turned away.

Although work was busy that day, she found her thoughts returning to the two words. As it turned out, it played on her mind for long after.

3

When she moved to the town of Glainkirk, having secured a coveted general practice partnership, never did Dr Cathy Moreland imagine that she might become so heavily involved in the crime of murder. The last two years in practice had undoubtedly been a strain. First, the death of one of her colleagues and then, a patient. As it turned out, she had been instrumental in uncovering the perpetrator in each case. The incidents were unrelated, but both had taken their toll on the fragile GP.

Cathy sighed. She swept a strand of hair from her lips and glanced in the rearview mirror before signalling to turn right. It was some time since she had been up this way, although, of course, she knew the catchment area quite well having worked there for some five years now. Most of the patients she saw were in Glainkirk itself, but being a market town, some were out in the sticks. She rather enjoyed the rural home visits if time wasn't too pressured. Admittedly, she could attend probably three patients in town, in the time it took her to do one in the country, but she always found escaping the bustle beneficial.

Being mid-January, the hedges that lined the roads were

sparse. Come springtime, it would look quite different. In the fields on either side of where she was now, the farmers might graze their cattle. Cathy found it cheering to see the young animals out with the sun on their backs. It signified a change for better things to come. She cast her eyes across the now desolate land. The empty fields seemed to go on forever. The vastness only punctuated by wooded copses and the sweeping line of tumbledown barbed-wire and hedge. It had already been a harsh winter and they were only now coming out the other side. Still, in the mornings, there was a hard frost underfoot.

Despite the blast of hot air from her car heater, Cathy shivered. She glanced down at the printed sheet that lay on the passenger seat. By the name of the house, she expected something grand. She'd not seen this gentleman before. Usually, James, her senior partner, dealt with him, but James was off work this week. She had locums covering his shifts, but it wasn't the same. Locums took an eternity to get to grips with the practice's particulars. Home visits, even routine ones, seemed to take them twice as long. She would be glad when James returned the week after next.

Although this had been a particularly strenuous one, it seemed that nowadays, every week merged into the following one. She had seen a brief chink in the monotony when she rekindled a friendship with someone she had known years ago, but things had gone a bit quiet as far as that was concerned. She couldn't blame him. The rigours of the job meant that she rarely finished on time, and when she did, she often took the work home. Recently, she had resorted to doing paperwork at her kitchen table on her days off, but her inability to switch off mentally was more of a problem. Many a night, she lay awake worrying about her patients and wondering if she had done the right thing. It was par for the course really. The job was well known for its uncertainties. If you couldn't cope with that, then you made a very poor doctor indeed. Cathy wondered how successful she was in this respect.

Over the years, she had wished she was more self-assured. Her closest friend from medical school, Suzalinna, now a consultant in accident and emergency, seemed to manage the balance just fine. In reality, the stakes were far greater for her friend. When people were wheeled into her department, it often fell to the consultant in charge to make a decisive call about treatment. The junior staff looked to Suzalinna for guidance and strong leadership. Cathy knew that her friend rarely wavered. If only she had the same resilience.

As she drove, Cathy grimaced. Of course, the imminent revalidation only made the situation worse. She knew it had to be done. These were the hoops through which she had to jump, along with all her fellow general practitioner colleagues. However, what was different in her case, was the added checking up. Her own GP, along with her psychiatrist, wrote three-monthly reports detailing occupational health of her progress. It was ridiculous really, to be so anxious about the thing every time. Cathy knew that if there was a problem, her doctor would speak to her first. Still, the threat of her fitness to practise being in question hung heavily. How simple life had been before. She wished she'd not taken her mental health for granted. Bipolar disorder in anyone might be life-altering, but for a doctor, it was unquestionably disastrous.

So much had changed since her extended time off work. Cathy shook her head. The confusion, the fear. She wouldn't allow herself to go through it all again. But that was what the psychiatrist had warned her of. A quiet life, he had recommended and when she had rolled his eyes, he had remained serious. No excitement. None at all, or risk heading back to hospital. Cathy knew that another relapse would undoubtedly put an end to her career. She had already tested her partner

James to the limit. She felt that she had let him and her patients down. James had been hugely understanding. He had covered for her, but he had also made it clear that they couldn't go on like that. It was unsafe for the patients; it was unhealthy for the partnership entirely.

Cathy wondered if James would have been as keen to take her on as junior partner had he known what was coming. She worried about the stress she had put on the practice as a whole, but primarily, she was troubled about James. He had borne the brunt. She knew that although he was incredibly discreet, he now kept a close eye on how she was. It had taken him this long to take a full two weeks off work since she had returned. She had blamed herself for his need to stay close, just in case something went wrong, but there was more to it than that.

'A regular one-week break is fine,' he had repeatedly told her. 'What am I going to do with a fortnight, anyway?'

Cathy knew what he meant. They were both lonely in their own way and a long spell away from work might only accentuate the fact. Cathy was still to find someone to share her life with, but poor James had found and then lost his life-partner. She knew it pained him greatly, even after five years, to know that despite all of his training and decades of experience, he had failed to spot the early signs of ovarian cancer in his wife. A tragedy it had been, but when he announced that he was taking two weeks holiday this time, Cathy's eyes had lit up with enthusiasm. She had heard mention of 'Elaine' more than once and hoped with all her heart that James might spend some of his well-earned break with this new and happy distraction. When he left the practice on Friday, Cathy had gently teased him.

'Don't get into mischief,' she said, and James had smiled and nodded.

'You, look after the place. I expect all the lab results to be kept up to date, and make a start on the insurance claims while I'm away.'

Cathy laughed. 'I'll be too busy policing the bloody locums.' But secretly, she wanted nothing more than to have James return to find the practice in excellent order, perhaps better than when he had left. She smiled as she thought of her senior partner.

And then suddenly, brought unceremoniously back the present, she jumped in fright and stamped hard on the brake pedal.

'Blast!'

There was a flapping of brown feathers and she waited for the thump. It didn't come, but as she tried to avoid the bird, the car swerved dangerously across the tarmac, its wheels sliding on the still-frosty surface. She struggled to maintain control and jammed the brakes too hard. The car juddered as its traction control attempted to kick in. She had the sickening realisation of what was about to happen only seconds before it did. She braced herself for the inevitable impact. The hedge was upon her. Thankfully, the collision was jarring but not great. The car came to an abrupt halt and everything that had been loud was then still. Cathy was aware of her own breathing. It came in shallow gasps as she fought back the unavoidable sting of tears. Just the shock. Stop being foolish. But the thud of heart still beat deafeningly in her ears for some minutes after.

The driver's side was higher up than it should be. The entire car was at a dreadful angle. Cathy swore and felt better for it. She knew that to get out of this predicament would be both diffi-cult and costly. What a bloody idiot she had been. If she'd just hit the damn pheasant instead of swerving, she would still be on her way to her patient. Instead, she was sitting in a ditch. Thank God she hadn't been going any faster. Her hands had been gently resting on the steering wheel, but looking down, she saw them now gripping it tightly. She forced her wrists to relax. Her arms ached. Her hands, as she opened them, were shaking.

She must get out. The car was still partially on the road and she would be in danger if another vehicle suddenly rounded the corner. Her seatbelt was tricky. She was too shaken to think to turn the engine off, but instead, opened the car door and scrambled out. The wheels on the passenger side were deep in the ditch. Cathy almost fell to her knees as she tried to stand. Ridiculous. And all this over a bloody pheasant. Thinking only now of the bird, she walked to the front of the bonnet. There was no sign.

'One of us had a lucky day then,' Cathy said sardonically.

She dialled the practice number on her mobile. It was Michelle who picked up.

'Oh goodness,' the receptionist said. 'Poor thing. And you're alright, other than a bit shaken?'

'I'm fine, but I can't see how I'll get to this visit now. Can you call and apologise for me? It was a routine one. I'll get there tomorrow.'

'Well, I'll not promise if your car's in a ditch,' Michelle said, laughing. 'What about afternoon surgery? Shall I move a few onto the locums, or put them off too?'

Cathy looked up and saw the slow approach of a tractor. She raised a hand and waved. The rumble of the approaching engine made it hard to hear. She returned to her mobile and shouted into it.

'Don't move anyone, Michelle. I'll be there one way or another, I promise. I'm not going to let anyone down.'

4

Gregory Warrender was a stocky sort of a man. His face generally held an expression of baffled ill-temper even when at rest. Life, on the whole, hadn't turned out as Gregory had wished. At the age of twenty-two, he had failed to impress his employers and had languished in a position far below his capability. Time and again, he had spoken to the estate manager about a promotion, if only just in title. This he knew, would have made all the difference to his wife anyway. He had been working for Dewhurst for such a long time now. How did Adam think he felt being on the same level as some of the seventeen-year-olds?

Adam had scoffed. 'If it's more money you're wanting out of Mr Dewhurst, you know you're going to struggle. You're already onto a good thing anyway. Think of the house, the Christmas bonuses. You could make more if you agreed to do the added shoots.'

Gregory had grunted and returned to expertly unwrapping a bale of treated straw with the prong on the front loader. Bloody cheek it was, and it was fine for Adam to be smug. He was in the old man's pocket. Gregory had noticed Mr Dewhurst slapping him on the back after the last pheasant shoot. Horrible, tweedy sport, Gregory had always thought. Unnecessary and barbaric. They had that smarmy gamekeeper Kenneth rearing the daft, feckless birds, actually hand-feeding them, and then, with little chance of escape, they were rounded up. Gregory knew that the idiots who came to shoot paid good money to be part of it. Either that or they were invited by Mr Dewhurst personally. By the time they headed off in their chauffeured Land Rovers, the majority of them were half-cut, God alone knew how they were allowed to handle a gun when they certainly wouldn't have been legal to drive. Many of the birds weren't killed outright. Mutilated and left to bleed into the mouths of Adam Foster's pack of nasty spaniels. Gregory shook his head in disgust.

As it happened, to appease his wife, Gregory had agreed to help at a few shoots this season, but the way the people spoke to you was outrageous. Thought they were above manners, most of them. He'd said this to Adam once. 'Bit sensitive, aren't we?' he had mocked. 'The man you were with today made his first million by the age of twenty-five. Sorry mate,' he had laughed. 'Completely different league, and yes, if he wants to talk down to you a bit, I'll not be stopping him.'

He'd never been fond of Adam. Fingers in too many pies, that one. Not to be trusted. He spoke to the farmhands like he was one of them when the fancy took him, but they all knew it wasn't the case. If Mr Dewhurst knew what an idle manager he had, he'd be less inclined to go slapping him on the back. Inwardly, Gregory seethed at the injustice of it all. Who was doing the real work, the manual labour?

As he reversed the tractor that afternoon, Gregory felt the anger simmer once again. His meaty hands grasped the steering wheel and he cursed under his breath. His face took on the look of a hungry bulldog whose bowl had been left empty for far too long. Of course, if it hadn't been for Fiona's constant needling, it might not have mattered quite so much. All she spoke about was climbing the damn social ladder these days.

Gregory shook his head in self-pity. Catching the train to that bloody office. Her earnings also gave him grave concern. It wasn't right for her to be bringing in more than him. So much had changed since she had left her job at the chippie. Admittedly, she had always told him it was a stop-gap and he had gone along with it as such, naively hoping that she might change her mind and even fall pregnant within the first year of marriage. At least then she might have settled down. It was much the same with cows. After their first calf, they were notoriously more placid. But instead of settling, Fiona had secured a job as an office assistant for Greysons, the road developers. Gregory had no idea what an office assistant really did. He assumed, photocopying. Hardly what you would call real work.

But that wasn't the half of it when it came to Fiona. He'd seen a change in her these past few months, playing up to the new gamey Kenneth. Thought he was stupid, probably, the pair of them. The lad parking his pickup right outside their house for all to see and carrying on like it was the most natural thing in the world. In Gregory's mind, men and women did not have simple friendships. Fine for Fiona to have her silly female friends at work, but to tell him that he was overreacting about her association with the bloody gamekeeper was pushing it.

Gregory tutted and the engine to his tractor roared as his foot depressed the accelerator. Sometimes when she came home in the evening, he was sure that she looked at him in a sneering, disappointed sort of way. That sister of hers was always on the phone, egging her on too. The whole family had never taken to him. He had tried to make an effort, really, he had, but when all was said and done, they both knew that the marriage had been a farce from the very start.

He cast his mind back. When they first met, he had of course known that she was a townie, but she had been so interested in the cattle. Many a weekend, she had been content to sit in the cab while he saw to the beasts. During calving, she had even made him an extra piece to have in the tractor in case he would have to stay late. But it had all changed, that was for sure.

Gregory's grip on the steering wheel slackened as he watched his favourite cow nodding slowly towards him. Her legs were partly obscured by the deep, golden straw which he had freshly lain in the run to the court yesterday morning. As she came towards the tractor at the entrance to the barn, she lowered her head. Her belly was ripe and it swung with a gentle, hypnotic rhythm. Only ten days until she would be due, he guessed. Likely as not, she'd do it alone and without the need of his help. A fine mother she had been to her calves over the years. He'd even put a rejected twin beside her the previous winter. She'd taken the scrawny thing on as her own. Gregory, despite his disgust at the injustice of it all, could not deny that he lived for these moments with his cows. Reliable, that's what they were. You knew where you were with them. You got the odd skittish one, of course. Those rarely made much of motherhood and ended up going to the fattening folk down the road, and a good thing too. No point in breeding again from them. Kindest thing was to send them away and be done with it.

If only life was as simple with women. But things might well be on the change. He had been turning things over in his mind for some time now. Especially since that morning's row with Fiona. Gregory snorted. Stupid; that's what they all thought of him. If Fiona and her stuck-up friends knew the truth they would be laughing on the other side of their faces. So would that bloody Adam Foster too, and Mr Dewhurst with his damn shooting parties.

A slow smile spread across Gregory's face. He touched the peak of his cap, sitting it more firmly on his perspiring head. Yes. If they knew, they'd be less likely to sneer, that was for sure.

---

athy smiled at the young woman before her. She was slight and quite pretty but her almond-shaped eyes had a somewhat nervous look about them.

'So how long would you say this has been going on?' Cathy asked.

The woman scrunched up her nose. 'It must be about a month, not more. The skin,' she continued, raising the sleeve of her blouse to further her point. 'That's been going on the longest. My face is bad too. I shouldn't have put on foundation really today, but I couldn't leave the house looking all blotchy, could I?'

Cathy nodded slightly. 'You mentioned your hair, Fiona? Can you tell me a little about that and any other symptoms? Tiredness, that sort of thing?'

The girl leaned forward. 'Look,' she said and pressed her parting flat for her doctor to see.

Cathy shifted in her seat and peered into the girl's hair. She wasn't convinced she saw anything, certainly no suggestion of alopecia. 'Just a few more general questions,' she said sitting back once more. 'Has there been any change in your mood or your weight?'

The girl looked affronted and shook her head.

'I know the questions sound odd, but I'm trying to build up a picture of things, you see? If it was just the dry skin, that would be a different matter, but the hair loss that you've noticed too, that can sometimes indicate something else. Have you been feeling unusually hot or cold recently?'

The girl snorted. 'Well, it's always cold in the house. The heating's been playing up dreadfully. Absolutely freezing sometimes. I've been going to bed early to get under the duvet.'

'And you live at …' Cathy turned to the computer screen and scanned the girl's notes.

'Glainkirk farm cottages. Yes, up at the big estate. My husband looks after Mr Dewhurst's cattle for him. You're probably imagining a chocolate-box cottage. Well, it's not like that at all. I've been onto Greg about moving for months. My friend's husband's an estate agent. He's meant to be on the lookout on my behalf. I'm more of a townie, myself,' she confided. 'Oh, we don't own the place, obviously,' she went on. 'Just rented from the old man. Discounted due to the job.'

'I see. Don't they have someone to contact regarding maintenance?' Cathy asked as she quickly typed her findings into the notes section on her computer.

The other woman snorted. 'Adam Foster? Yes. He's the estate manager. My husband and he don't see eye to eye. Maybe I should have a word. I keep pestering Greg to speak to him about the house, but I'll bet he's not bothered. Perhaps I'll do it on the way home from work later. It was the same with the bloody mice. Greg took it upon himself to sort that out too rather than ask for pest control.'

'How are things at home?' Cathy asked, allowing her hands to drop from the keyboard. She studied the woman's face. 'You've only been married a year and a bit?'

Fiona looked away and then grimaced. 'Yes. Not great,' she

admitted. Her hands twisted in her lap. 'It's not been the easiest, to be fair. Maybe Mum was right. We're both very young. I got an office job at Greysons in Forkieth six months back. Greg wasn't happy about it. A dent to his ego, I think.' She rolled her eyes and grinned, but Cathy didn't smile.

'You've been having a few issues, arguments?'

The woman snorted. 'More than a few!' She seemed to be weighing up whether to say more and then she blurted it out. 'For a time, I wondered if he might actually be poisoning me! It's been playing on my mind a good bit. The hair and the skin, you see?' She laughed. 'I've been watching too many of those silly crime documentaries late at night.'

Cathy looked into the other woman's eyes. She hadn't failed to spot the mottled purple of what looked like a bruise on the inside of her wrist.

'I think poisoning is highly unlikely,' she said slowly. 'First, I tend to rule out the more obvious things, like thyroid problems, or anaemia.' She smiled. 'Are you sure there's nothing more? When someone, even jokingly, accuses their husband of something like that ...'

The girl shook her head. 'I'm being silly,' she said. 'Overactive imagination. I've always had one. That's what Mum would say anyway.'

Cathy smiled. 'As far as the skin and the hair are concerned, I think we'd better run a blood test just to check. It's really to rule out any underlying medical issue as I said. I see in your notes that there's no recorded family history of thyroid disease.'

The girl shook her head. 'There's nothing as far as I know.'

Cathy crossed the room to her sink and washed her hands. She'd take the blood sample herself rather than asking her to make an appointment with the nurse.

'Family in the area?' she asked as she continued to collect what she needed.

'Mum and sister. Dad died years ago.'

'Supportive?'

'Oh yes, and I have my friends too.'

Cathy nodded. At least this gave her some reassurance. 'If you roll up your sleeve, I'll do the bloods now.'

The bruise was revealed once more. Cathy wondered if it was a thumbprint. She hesitated.

'Oh, knocked myself,' Fiona said, seeming to realise.

'Right. You're not squeamish, are you?'

The girl laughed. 'Hardly. You can't be, living with a farmer.'

Cathy smiled. 'When you mentioned the mice, admittedly, it did make my toes curl.'

The girl seemed to relax for the first time during the consultation. She grinned. 'Mice! That's nothing. Honestly, it's been a steep learning curve since Greg and I met. Rats are what get me. Hate them, and of course, they're all over, being on a farm. I try not to think about it. Greg told me they had a bit of a problem with them a few years back. Thankfully, before my time,' she said. 'Got so bad the farmhands were going up to the cattle courts at night. Traps weren't keeping on top of them, so they were taking pop-shots.'

'Shooting rats?' Cathy asked, hardly able to hide her incredulity.

'Tell me about it. It's disgusting. You're better not knowing really. Rabbits are regular pests. I don't mind them so much. I'm not a fan of guns. The estate runs pheasant shoots in the winter. I hate the noise.'

'I wonder if it was someone from your husband's farm who got me out of a fix the other week,' Cathy said as she slipped the tourniquet over the girl's hand. She drew the elastic tight around her upper arm and set out her bottles and needle on a cardboard tray on the desk. 'I was doing a visit up in the area but a pheasant flew in front of the car and I swerved into a ditch,' she said. 'Had to flag down a tractor to pull me out. Lucky really,' she said. 'Could have been much worse. The car was pretty much undamaged. Here comes a sharp scratch,' she said as she rested the needle tip to a vein. The girl flinched slightly but didn't speak. The bottles filled quickly. 'There you are,' she said. 'That'll save you making another appointment with the nurse.' She unclicked the tourniquet and pushed a small wad of cotton wool to the woman's elbow. 'Press on that for a minute,' she said.

She began to label the bottles and as she did so, she continued to talk. 'I should have asked about your menstrual cycle,' she said. She glanced up and saw the woman's look of horror. 'Oh no, nothing worrying. I hope you're not offended. It's just that some medical conditions can affect your periods.'

The woman exhaled. 'I thought you were accusing me of being pregnant. No, there's not any change there. I'm always a bit all over the place as far as that's concerned.'

Cathy smiled. 'If there's anything unusual with the results, I'll get the girls at reception to give you a call.'

The other woman nodded and began to gather her things, scooping up her winter jacket that had fallen from the back of the chair onto the floor.

'If there's anything else ...' Cathy urged, but she was already heading to the door.

'No that's about all. Thanks for your time,' she said. 'You've been nice.'

When Cathy was alone once again, she sighed. Such a difficult consultation to get right. An unhappy marriage and a visible bruise on the woman's arm. It didn't sit well with her, especially when the conversation had turned to talk of poison, and worse still, guns. But perhaps she was being oversensitive. The woman had, after all, reassured her. She had friends and family around and had even said herself that she was probably being melodramatic.

Cathy tidied her desk and was about to call the next patient in when something the young woman had said came back to her. *I thought you were accusing me of being pregnant.* Accuse? What an odd choice of words. And even more so, for a married woman. Cathy shook her head. No, she decided, as she crossed the room, she had a feeling it might not be the last she saw of the girl Fiona Warrender.

Old Mr Dewhurst crossed to the window and looked out. The vast expanse of land was his family's and had been for generations. When his father had died, Glainkirk Estate had fallen to his older brother, but he had long since died. A freak accident after only living in the place for a matter of months. The corners of Mr Dewhurst's mouth, now wrinkled and thin, turned up in a sneer. A bloody disaster that would have been. In many ways, fate had taken its rightful course allowing him to inherit and take charge of the place.

He looked around the room dispassionately. Odd how little pleasure he gained from it these days. When once, he had revelled in the opportunity to stamp his mark, all he now saw were problems. To the inattentive eye, they might go unnoticed. The slightly discoloured patch in the top right-hand corner in the drawing-room, the peeling velvety paper by the door in the once-great hall.

Slowly, he turned and lowered himself into a chair. He had taken his eye off of things for too long perhaps. He looked up at the painting above in its gilt frame. A portrait of his great-grand-father. The old man looked back severely. Indeed, he might well not approve of things as they stood. Mr Dewhurst shook his head sadly. It was well-known that his ancestor had been frugal to the extreme. Others before him might have pawned off the family valuables in times of trouble, but he had refused. When Mr Dewhurst's grandfather had inherited, the place had been in some considerable disorder, but only, it seemed, because his predecessor had been living in a single room with his valuables around him for near enough ten years, refusing to waste money on the heating of the rest.

Mr Dewhurst sighed. He shifted his glasses off the bridge of his nose and rubbed the indentation. Times had changed. Replacing his spectacles, he reached to his top pocket and removed the piece of paper. He unfolded it and re-read it, wincing despite knowing the words almost by heart. Certainly, it was a sad state of affairs. He had let his guard down since Marjory's death. Now, he was in real difficulty. Mr Dewhurst shook his head in distaste. The very idea was abhorrent. Why had he entertained their advances in the first place? And now, they were rushing him. Mr Dewhurst disliked being hurried. It wasn't the way he worked.

The old man raised himself and, walking to the far window, looked out and along the wide, gravelled drive leading to the lodge. It had been an idyllic existence for many years. Or had it? In the background, there had perhaps always been an undercurrent of concern, even when Marjory was alive. They had swept a good deal under the carpet, undoubtedly. She had been more business-minded than him. And now, what was left? He had no son to pass the place to. Perhaps he was being pig-headed after all. If he agreed to their demands, all this would be over. The sleepless nights, the worrying ...

The old man turned on his heel, his face now emotionless, his eyes, hard.

'Time for a change,' he said quietly. 'Yes, perhaps it is time for a change.'

It was gone seven-forty-five. Rosemary spun on her heel and walked back along the platform. Stepping sideways to avoid a rather scruffy-looking man who was drinking from a polystyrene cup, she looked at the screen on her phone. Nothing. The tannoy crackled and informed her that the train approaching platform two was the seven-forty for Forkieth. The announcer then reeled off all of the minor stations at which the commuter train would stop. Where the hell was she?

Rosemary drew her jacket tightly around her waist as a sudden gust of wind buffeted her. She surveyed the car park. No vehicle was pulling in. When she had seen Fiona's bus come and go already without the girl on it, she had assumed she might still make it by catching a lift with someone from the farm.

Behind her, Rosemary heard the rails sing as the train neared. 'Come on,' she said under her breath, just as a set of headlights from an approaching car came into view. The car accelerated down the road towards the station, but at the round-about, where it should turn in, it continued. Damn. The silly girl was going to miss the train and possibly lose her job now. Well, it was her own fault. Rosemary had gone out of her way to help her get the position in the first place. It felt like a slap in the face after she had taken such trouble.

She had originally met Fiona when the other girl was serving in the local chip shop on Glainkirk High Street. Rosemary was not a regular and liked to keep an eye on her waistline anyway, but after a dreadful day at work, David had suggested she collect a fish supper for them both as she would be passing on the way home. A treat to cheer them both up, he had said when she called him on the way back. Rosemary didn't know why her husband needed cheering up. As far as she could tell, his life was enviably simple, working as a reasonably well-paid estate agent with few managerial worries. But not wanting to ruin the sentiment, she agreed.

Rosemary didn't take much notice of the girl serving her. She was the only customer in the shop and after placing her order, she sat on the tiled window ledge to wait. The smell of grease and vinegar clung to everything and she found herself wondering how the staff didn't end up with oily skin and lank hair. Rosemary looked out at the passing cars, their headlights catching the window as they passed. Other commuters making their way home. She sighed.

'Tough day?' the girl at the counter asked.

Rosemary turned, and for the first time, took in the smiling, impish-looking face. Rosemary judged that she must have only recently left school. She nodded. 'The worst. One of the office girls walked out yesterday. I'm PA to the managing director and have enough on my plate without the extra stress. I've been doing both her and my own work today. The boss wasn't best pleased, especially when we were in the middle of something important.'

The girl behind the counter grinned and gestured towards the back door. 'I know how you feel. They're too tight to employ extra here. It's quiet now, but on a Friday, it's chaos. I hate people having to wait, and if I'm hashed, I make mistakes. This was only meant to be a stop-gap for me as well. I'll only stay on working here because there's nothing else.'

Rosemary nodded in sympathy and stood by the counter now as the girl continued to turn the fish in the hot grill. Apparently happy with the colour of the fish, the girl selected two and placed them on the blank newsprint which lay in a neat stack in front of her. She shovelled her spatula deep into the trough of golden chips.

'Here you go,' she said. 'This'll cheer you up anyway. Salt and vinegar?'

Rosemary nodded.

The girl glanced over her shoulder as Rosemary dipped into her handbag to find her purse.

'On me,' she whispered.

'No, I can't,' Rosemary protested.

'Honestly,' the girl said, shaking her head. 'It's only a poke of chips.'

Rosemary remonstrated again and handed over the money. She thanked the girl profusely and left with the fish suppers. Her faith in humanity had been restored.

When she got home and told David about the happy encounter, he had snorted and told her she should have asked the chippie girl if she wanted the job going at her work. Rosemary had smiled, but the idea had, of course, stuck. After a week of relentlessly phoning around agencies and with still no sign of a replacement, she found herself in the chip shop once more with a proposition.

That had been six months ago. She'd not regretted her decision to approach Fiona so far, but now this ... Reluctantly, Rosemary turned from the road. It was too late. And of course, it looked bad on her also. She had recommended Fiona in the first place. She hated to disappoint Mr Greyson. The silly girl had let her down.

Along with the other commuters, she followed the crawling train, until the doors came level and the button saying 'open' flashed, allowing her to board. Rosemary found a seat to herself. She then arranged her things on the neighbouring one so that no-one might be tempted to join her. The carriage wasn't too busy anyway. Usually, she and Fiona would try for a table-seat, but there was no point if you were on your own. As the doors hissed shut, Rosemary watched the platform disappear. She reached again for her mobile. Still nothing. She should send a text and find out. In the six months or so of Fiona working with her, it was the third time she had failed to show. On the previous and most recent occasion, it had turned out that she had forgotten to tell her about a doctor's appointment. Well, that's what she had said anyway. Rosemary began to key in the message: 'Where on earth ...' and then, she was aware of someone standing by her shoulder. She turned in her seat and looked up.

'May I?' the lady asked, gesturing to the seat beside Rosemary.

Rosemary glanced across the aisle at the multitude of empty seats, but not wanting to make a fuss, she shifted her handbag to her knee and smiled slightly, returning to her mobile phone screen.

'Thank you,' the woman said, lowering herself into the seat and jogging Rosemary's elbow as she did so. 'I thought I recognised you from a couple of weeks ago.'

Rosemary, having sent her text message, looked at the woman properly and finally realised. 'Of course. You were on the train with us the other week,' she said.

The elderly woman nodded. 'You're alone today though?'

Rosemary snorted. 'I was just sending her a message. The

boss will be furious if she doesn't make it to work. Big day for us. Presentation to the financiers. Oh, not us,' Rosemary said hurriedly. 'I mean the company. No, Fiona and I are only glorified office-girls.'

'Even the smallest cogs,' the woman said, and Rosemary nodded.

'Exactly. Without us, it doesn't run, the whole place would grind to a halt.'

Rosemary glanced at her phone. The screen lit up and she read the message.

'Trouble?' her new travel companion asked.

'Slept in, apparently,' she said, clicking the phone off. 'I think she's trying to get someone to drive her now, but she'll be late. It will look dreadful.'

'You'll cover for her,' the woman said knowingly.

Rosemary smiled thinly. She supposed she would have to, but the elderly woman wasn't finished. 'She needs a bit of looking after anyway, your friend. I could tell that.'

Rosemary turned in her seat. 'Oh?' How do you mean?' she asked. 'Do you know Fiona then?'

'I don't know her at all,' the woman replied. 'But I don't need to. I hope you don't mind me saying,' she went on. 'It's just that I overheard. I've been kicking myself since for not saying anything at the time. She was talking about her husband that day and it made me think rather.'

Rosemary felt distinctly uncomfortable with the direction the conversation had taken. She shifted in her seat and glanced across the aisle, trying to recall what she and Fiona had said.

'I know it's not very British to start up a conversation with a stranger,' the old woman said. 'But I'd said to myself that if I met the pair of you again, I'd say something. I catch this train up every Thursday, you see? Robert, that was my husband, he's buried in the churchyard in Forkieth and it's my weekly visit.'

'I'm sorry,' Rosemary said automatically.

'Oh goodness, don't be,' the woman beside her said. 'It's been the making of me. I wish it could have happened sooner.'

Rosemary gaped.

'Not a nice thing to say, I realise,' the elderly woman said with a smile. 'But we were wholly incompatible from the start. Rough, he was. He spoke down to me, and I ended up making do and regretting the day we met.'

Rosemary shook her head, still unsure of what to say.

'I suppose that's what I had wanted to say to your friend,' she went on. 'I heard what she was saying, you understand? About her husband. I know you'll think it a presumption, but I'd hate to see someone else wasting her life like myself.' The elderly woman's eyes creased as she smiled to herself. 'In many ways, I was lucky. It was different in my day. You married the person your parents wanted you to marry. You did it to please them, or sometimes,' she said, smiling more broadly, 'to spite them if you wanted to leave home.'

Rosemary found herself smiling back.

'Back then, you did just 'make do' when things weren't so rosy,' the woman continued. 'The aversion didn't run so deep. Oh, I know there's divorce nowadays as a get-out. Funnily, it isn't always so simple. Your friend though. I worry about resentment. Love can turn to bitterness far sooner than you think. When resentment sets in, it's incredibly dangerous.'

Rosemary found herself dumbstruck, and for the rest of the journey, she sat in silence, watching the fields and houses flash past without notice. She was glad when they arrived at her station and she was able to alight into the fresh air. As she walked the short distance to work, she pulled at the collar on her felt jacket and glanced up. The sky, that had initially seemed bright when she had left the house that morning, had taken on an imposing quality. A storm was coming. That was for sure.

8

'That's fine, you can sort yourself out again,' Cathy said, replacing the sphygmomanometer in her bag and jotting down the third reading.

The elderly gentleman tugged at his rolled-up sleeve, loosening the folds and allowing the shirt to fall to his wrist. 'Well?' he asked. 'What's the verdict? Am I done for?'

Cathy smiled, but she wasn't happy. 'Still too high,' she said. 'You've been taking the tablets as prescribed?'

He nodded.

It was four days following her first attempt to visit Mr Dewhurst. His demeanour was at first upright and rather severe, but he broke type and chuckled when she told him the reason for her aborted mission the week before. 'Blasted pest they are, but we'll get a few off the roads soon enough. A big shoot in a week or so,' he explained. 'I'm glad someone came to your aid though. Probably one of our lot. They're up and down the road seeing to the fencing just now. Never-ending business,' he sighed.

'It must be a big job managing the place,' Cathy said. She had never driven up to the estate before and wasn't sure how much land belonged to the family. The house itself was sprawling and as she had entered, she wondered how the old man coped living there alone with, apparently, only a housekeeper.

He sighed again. 'I'm getting old.'

'You have people working for you? You mentioned the farmhands and the lady who showed me up ...'

'Mrs Mackenzie? She's alright. Been with us for nearly thirty years. My wife didn't much warm to her. Too domineering. She has her ideas and won't allow you to talk her around. My wife used to threaten to sack her. "We're meant to be the ones in charge," she used to say.' The old man smiled. He leaned in as if sharing a great secret 'The truth is that I don't mind letting her boss me a little. In some ways, it's a comfort since Marjory passed away.' He sighed and turned to look out through the vast window at the countryside that surrounded them. 'Oh, I've other people looking after the land,' he continued. 'Most of that side of things is down to the estate manager.'

'I'll listen to your heart if I may,' Cathy quickly said, as she saw that he was beginning to put on his tweed jacket. 'Sorry,' she said.

He raised his hands in acceptance and began to undo the top buttons on his shirt, his hands trembled slightly and Cathy wondered if it was due to the effort or the conversation they had just had.

She leant closer, listening to the lub-dup, rhythmic beat. 'If I might look at your ankles too? It's to check for swelling. Dr Longmuir may have mentioned that the tablets he prescribed can sometimes do that.' She ran her fingers over the man's skin, depressing it and checking for any puffiness.

'I'm still concerned,' she admitted having finished. 'Your heart sounds are fine and there's no significant ankle oedema, but the blood pressure hasn't come down at all as I had hoped it might. Have you had any other symptoms? Headaches, blurred vision? Dr Longmuir noted that you were complaining of migraines when he first saw you. That was a couple of weeks back now. Has that still been a bother?'

Mr Dewhurst shook his head.

'You can dress again.' She began to tidy her things. 'The tablets that Dr Longmuir prescribed?' she asked. 'Have you had any side-effects at all? Light-headedness, dizziness when getting up in the morning?'

'Not that I've noticed. I'm too busy to be worrying about that.'

Cathy nodded, weighing up the choice of increasing the current antihypertensive medication or adding in a different one. 'I think, as the blood pressure is so high,' she decided, 'we'll add in something new. Funnily enough, it might well sort out swollen ankles if you do start to develop them, but it might also make you need to go to the toilet more often. Oh, I know,' she said to the old man's frown. 'But I can't leave you like this. You're at risk of having a stroke if you continue this way.'

She tidied her stethoscope into her bag, folding the rubber tubing over and around the earpieces. 'You mentioned a shoot coming up?'

'Now, Doctor, please don't spoil the little enjoyment I have.'

'I'm not telling you that you can't go, I'm just –'

'You're just advising me that I shouldn't shoot a gun because if I have a stroke or a heart attack while doing so and acciden-tally kill my estate manager, you'll be liable?'

Cathy laughed. 'Oh, my goodness, no. Look, I'm not your keeper. High blood pressure isn't a contraindication for shooting pheasants. I think however, that keeping things like that to a minimum is advisable. Now,' Cathy continued, straightening up from her bag. 'I understand that Dr Longmuir usually pops in on the way past. I would like to check your blood pressure again, perhaps next week. Is there any way you could make it into the surgery to see me next time?'

'Can't shoot, but I'm alright to drive?' he mocked. 'No, you don't need to explain. You're a busy woman, I can see that. I'll come to you from now on. Don't want you crashing into a ditch again, now do we?'

Cathy glanced at him, unsure if he really was teasing. 'Your new prescription will be ready for collection later today,' she said.

They walked together to the door in silence, but when they reached it, he turned to her. 'Dr Longmuir told me about you,' he said. 'He holds you in very high regard.'

Cathy's cheeks flushed.

'Oh, he was quite genuine in his praise. Told me you'd be an excellent fill-in while he was off this week. Perhaps I'll not want to return to his care. I had heard that you had been involved with sorting out the little indiscretion at your work.'

Cathy grimaced. Hardly an indiscretion having a member of the practice murdered, but she knew what he meant. 'Anyway,' she said as they stood on the stone steps outside. 'Next week?'

He bowed his assent.

Her car was parked to the far side of the sweeping driveway, and as she retreated, she was aware of the old man's eyes following her. Lonely sort of existence, Cathy thought. She glanced back and he was still standing in the doorway.

9

If it hadn't been for having a hobby during his first year of marriage, Gregory might well have resorted to murder by now. As he tramped the furrowed land that late Sunday afternoon, he cast his mind back to a story his mother had once told him about a distant relative. Perhaps the family trait was present in him also. If he remembered rightly, his mother had said that the man hadn't been so distant as he had originally thought. Mad, she had told him when the subject came up. How they had ended up talking about it, Gregory couldn't imagine, but he had pressed his mother, being in his teenage years and keen to hear a gory tale. 'Mad. Crazy mad,' she had repeated, as she folded the enormous pile of sheets on the kitchen table.

'But what happened?' Gregory had asked, only knowing half the story.

His mother paused, and then seemingly deciding that he was old enough to hear, she continued. 'You never met him of course,' she said. 'I'd barely started stepping out with your father back then. He was settled, and the family hadn't seen him for near-on a month, as it turned out.'

Young Gregory waited, leaning on the countertop beside the stove.

'Dreadful for everyone concerned,' his mother said, shaking her head. 'Nearly ended my own mother. It was her younger brother, after all. I asked her about it a few years later and she said he'd never shown any sign of it. Madness, I mean. Dead, they were found,' she explained, glancing at him. 'God knows, the place must've been stinking. It was near-enough a week they'd lain there, in his cottage, the pair of them.'

Gregory still didn't speak.

'Shot,' his mother said shortly and she slapped the pile of sheets with the palm of her hand. 'He killed her; his wife, and then it seems, regretting it, he turned the gun on himself. Couldn't happen these days. More careful with their gun laws and all that nonsense now, I suppose. Dreadful all the same. A big embarrassment for the family. Weren't meant to talk about it at all. Hushed up.'

The then-young Gregory smiled slowly. 'Perhaps I'll do the same myself when I get wed,' he said, purely to vex his mother. She had flicked a pillowcase at him and told him to get out of her kitchen, or she'd see his father took a pop at him instead of the rabbits that evening.

Strange, thinking back to it now, Gregory considered as he paused and hovered the detector over the ground. He moved the machine this way and that, his mother's story now forgotten. He was sure it was here the last time he had been out. There had been several interesting areas at this side of the field, and he had been keen to come back and investigate. If bloody Adam Foster knew what he was doing, he'd probably have a fit. Gregory smirked. It was a free country and he'd not found anything valuable yet. That, he hoped was soon to change.

He paused, sure he was in the right place and then something caught his eye from far across the field, the reflection of sunlight on something, perhaps glass. Gregory straightened up and peered into the wooded area in the distance. It was where many of the pheasants were roosting currently, a haven before the shoots in the coming weeks. He was positive that there had been a light, but perhaps he had imagined it. Too jumpy, he thought ruefully.

He returned to the ground before him, swinging the detector this way and that. A smile twitched on Gregory's thin lips. Imagine if he did find something significant. What would Adam Foster have to say to that? Not just Adam, but Mr Dewhurst. Of course, if he found anything on Dewhurst's estate, there could possibly be some dispute over ownership. Gregory wasn't stupid though. He'd already planned for that. If he discovered anything of value, he'd not be showy. He'd keep it quiet, to himself. Even Fiona need not know immediately. This idea pleased him perhaps more greatly than the thought of outwitting his employers. Yes, imagine knowing that he sat on some substantial find, a small fortune, and all the while, his wife was beavering away at her silly office job, lording it up, like she was better than him. Laughing at him with her fancy friends and that dreadful gamekeeper Kenneth. What amusement it might give him, to listen to her talking down to him, while only he knew.

The detector whined and then a constant beep sounded. He had been right. Laying the sensor down carefully by the verge, Gregory took a small trowel from his jacket pocket and began to gently scrape the ground.

10

'Where have you been?' David asked without looking at her.

The television was on and Rosemary grimaced as she came into the room.

'Don't start,' she sighed and then raising her voice so it could be heard: 'I told you before I had to pop into work. It's been so busy this week, I couldn't stand the thought of tomorrow morning. All the mail mounted up on my desk,' She picked up the remote and pressed the volume button. David tutted. 'Anyway,' she said, ignoring him, 'it's fine now.' She dropped the remote and the car keys on the chair beside him. 'I filled it up for you,' she said.

He didn't acknowledge her gesture and returned his attention to the football, which seemed to be at a critical point. Rosemary watched her husband as he leaned forward, gripping the edge of the chair. 'Come on, come on,' he urged the screen. 'Jesus!' he shouted and fell back in disgust as the player missed the opportunity to score.

Rosemary turned in the doorway but he shifted to address her once more. 'Work though? On a Sunday, Rose? I hope Alfie-

Bloody-Greyson knows how lucky he is to have you. Our lot wouldn't expect it. I told you before, if it gets too much, we'd take you on. I think you'd secretly rather like to work for me.'

Rosemary didn't answer. Her husband had indeed said this many times before. She removed her heels and swung them from her hand. A clod of mud fell from one of the heels onto the carpet. She sighed and retraced her steps, seeing a line of earth she had brought in. Rosemary went to the kitchen. Armed with a sponge and a basin of soapy water, she painstakingly dabbed, paring back the fibres until they were back to their original colour. David seemed oblivious.

Still crouched in the hall, she heard him roaring with delight in the living room, evidently, his team had scored. Thank God for that. She'd need to get the evening meal on really. She had wondered if David might have sorted something while she was out, but it seemed not. It didn't matter. She had planned a pasta dish at some point this week, and for ease, it would be tonight.

'If I do dinner in forty?' she asked, coming through once more.

David looked up at her, beaming. 'Come here,' he said and stretched out an arm. As she neared, he grabbed her, pulling her down on top of him. 'Sorry for being a pig.'

'David, my skirt,' she laughed.

'Sod the skirt. Oh Rose,' he said, looking at her properly for the first time. 'You are rather wonderful.'

She pushed herself back and looked at him. 'All because your team scored?'

'You know it's not that. I got a call earlier, while you were out. I swear, things are on the up. If I manage to pull this off, I promise we'll move away from Glainkirk, perhaps to a larger house in the country.'

Rosemary's face fell. 'Not this again. We're quite content

here. We only moved a year ago, anyway. Look, I'm happy you're making progress at work …'

He shook his head. 'You've no idea what I mean, really Rosemary,' he said, holding her waist tightly. His expression was intense and she couldn't help laughing.

'Seriously, this could be big, really big, Rose. I'm not talking about a small-scale development. This could push the company far.'

'You're a land and estate agent, David, not some business tycoon.'

'They're crying out for this kind of a deal, I tell you. I've done all the groundwork myself. It's been all me, no-one else involved, just me. If I see it through smoothly …' He looked up at her, his eyes almost frightening with passion.

Rosemary watched his pupils constrict. Blood rushed to her face and glanced over his shoulder at the clock. 'I'd better get the dinner on,' she said and shifted off his knee.

Leaving the room, she felt sick. Out of loyalty, she couldn't contradict him, but she knew only too well that it was nonsense. Even if he did pull it off, it was unlikely to provide them the kind of security that he hoped. That was David all over though.

Rosemary thought of her parents, miles away in London. Her father was now semi-retired. A real businessman, the old-fashioned sort. Instinctive and sharp. When she had introduced David to them, he had been oblivious to how foolish he had seemed. The family had all watched on. Her mother's face had been a picture. David had pandered and faltered his way in conversation, overcomplimenting Rosemary's father on his commercial acumen. Rosemary grimaced at the memory. Perhaps it was because of it, that she had married David in the end. None had been more mortified than Rosemary herself at his naive behaviour, but despite coming from an affluent background, she couldn't abide snobbery of any sort. It was months since she and her parents had last spoken. A great disappointment her decision had been to both of them.

Rosemary filled the kettle and then began to assemble the ingredients she would need. What he didn't realise was that he was a small fish in a very big pond. She had tried to explain but still, he persisted. That was David though. But he wasn't just a daydreamer. It was more dangerous than that. He was delusional. Sometimes, Rosemary wasn't sure what to believe when he said things to her now.

Through in the other room, she heard him whistling to himself. Rosemary's stomach lurched. It was painful to witness his simplicity. It almost made her feel guilty.

11

I t was gone five o'clock when he finished. Gregory wrapped his metal-detector in a towel that sat in the back of the jeep. He removed the trowel from his pocket and wiped the metal surface clean with the sleeve of his jacket and placed it in the boot. From his other pocket, he retrieved his finds. Two coins this time. He was now in no doubt at all that he would find more. He had already polished the surface of both and, in the dying sunlight, the bronze hue took on a deep warmth. He studied them again now, running his grubby thumb over the dented surface. Things were undoubtedly going to change on Glainkirk Farm Estate, that was for sure. Smiling, he carefully rewrapped both in a handkerchief and pocketing them, got in the car. He had no concerns about Fiona. Even if she was suspicious enough to go through his things, she wouldn't have a clue what she was looking at.

Gregory started the engine. Undoubtedly, living on the estate was a bonus but it did mean that his work was rarely far from his mind. He looked out onto the field that would, in a month or two, sustain his entire herd of cattle. The grass was still to come through after the harsh season. It had been a wet winter and this had only served to leach the vital minerals from the soil allowing the nutrients to run off the gentle gradient. A fertiliser would be needed. That was if Dewhurst agreed to fork out. He'd been funny over money recently. Gregory had blamed it as much on Adam. He was the gatekeeper to all the estate finances. Adam had been unwilling to even talk about fertilisers or pesticides this year. Complete madness, Gregory had thought. If they allowed the land to go, even for a single year, to save money, they'd be paying for it for many more to come in loss of crop yield. Gregory wondered if Mr Dewhurst had lost his enthusiasm for the farm as a business. He was after quick money, more than likely, and farming didn't offer fast rewards. Gregory had asked Adam to consider proposing a scheme he had come up with, of drying their own hay. Too much hassle, Adam had said. Silage was simple and quick. This hay nonsense was a waste of resources and time. Gregory hadn't bothered to argue. He knew plenty of farms across the county that did an excellent trade in forage once the storage was organised. All it took was a bit of outlay in setting the thing up. A shed for storage, and if they wanted to do it well, a drying system. The better the quality of the hay, the more they could charge for it. Gregory knew one farm that sold small, square bales for seven pounds. Seven pounds! But there was no point in arguing.

As he drove, Gregory looked left and across the fields. The great house belonging to the Dewhursts came into view through a thicket of trees. God alone knew how they managed to heat the sprawling place. Things were hard enough to keep on top of in his own modest cottage. Gregory slowed as he approached the end of the drive leading up to the main gates. At the bottom was the estate office where Adam worked. Adam himself didn't live on-site but instead chose to stay in town. Gregory didn't know what the other man's home looked like. More than likely it was swish. That was how Adam was.

He was almost at the end of the long, sweeping drive now and he happened to glance again up the line of trees that flanked it. He was sure he'd seen something in one of the office windows moving. Gregory slowed and then brought the jeep to a standstill. Perhaps he'd been mistaken. He thought again of the flash of sunlight landing on something earlier. Was he going mad today? He remained still and watched. There was no sign of Adam's car if he had decided to come in on the weekend to catch up with paperwork. No-one should be in the estate office on an early Sunday evening.

Gregory sat, the car stationary, his eyes fixed on the office window. In truth, he was in no hurry to return home. Fiona only had time for frozen meals these days. No doubt he'd simply be reheating in the microwave something she had defrosted earlier. He had almost decided that he had been mistaken and that again, the illusion had been a trick of the light as it fell on the glass. But just as he was about the release the handbrake and move off, he saw something again. A shadow moving from within the office and a flash of light. His heart quickened. If the person inside had a legitimate reason to be there, why wasn't there a car outside? More importantly, why was the place in darkness and the person within using a torch?

Gregory drove the jeep up onto the grass verge and silenced the engine. He was still a good fifty metres from the turning, and then another fifty to the office itself. He shut the door to his car quietly and crossed the gravelled path, his feet crunching on the loose stones. As he approached, he had little idea of what he was going to do if he did discover a burglar. This thought made him pause. He retreated and from the boot took a spade that he had brought from the garden shed that afternoon in case his detector had found something requiring deeper excavation.

He was unsure if there was anything of value in the office that weekend. He knew that Adam paid many of the employees cash-in-hand weekly. Gregory had been on a monthly contract for just over six months. Adam had peddled this to him as a step up the ladder, setting him apart from the manual labourers. Gregory had fallen for this until, returning home to tell Fiona, she had scoffed and said it was probably a time-saving thing, and that employers were all being forced away from casual contracts, it was the law. Gregory approached cautiously once again. Imagine if he caught someone mid-robbery.

He was now level with the estate office. The door was closed. He tried the handle, balancing the spade in his other hand carefully so as not to make a noise and alert the possible intruder. The door opened without a sound, but from within the building, Gregory could hear what sounded like a drawer being closed. He stood motionless in the small reception area, listening. Papers were being leafed through and then he heard a man's hollow cough. Not knowing if he should just open the door to the office and surprise the intruder, he rested the spade at his feet. His heart was beating loudly now in his ears. So loudly in fact, that he almost missed the sound of footsteps. The intruder was crossing the room. They were coming towards the door. In a moment of panic, Gregory ducked behind a gun cabinet by the wall. His breathing was shallow as he prepared to pounce.

The door to Adam's office opened and the intruder emerged. Gregory held his breath. But to his amazement, he saw that it was none other than Adam himself. Gregory did a double-take when he saw the man because instead of wearing his usual smart shirt and tie, he was dressed in jeans and a dirty-looking black jumper. His face too was different. He was not cleanshaven but had allowed a shadow of stubble to accumulate and his expression was of deathly seriousness. Gregory wasn't sure why he didn't come out of his hiding place at that point. Nothing could have been simpler than explaining that he had been there as he'd thought there was a robbery in progress and had come to prevent the estate being looted. But instead, he froze, his body pressed hard against the wall, hoping that whatever else happened, Adam would not look to his right as he exited the building.

Gregory noticed a brown envelope in Adam's hand. The man looked shifty to the extreme. Thankfully, as he passed, Adam didn't see him. He pulled the door shut and Gregory exhaled in relief. But then he heard a key being turned. Gregory knew that to dash to the door and hammer on it, was impossible. Adam looked in no humour to find that he had been spied on. Instead, his mind racing, Gregory stepped out from behind the cabinet. He waited until he was sure he was safe to do so, and then peered through the blinds covering the reception window. Adam was nowhere to be seen, but Gregory heard a car engine start, and then Adam's car emerged from behind the building and the estate manager left.

Gregory was dumbfounded. What on earth had Adam been playing at, sneaking around the place? And why had he parked his car out of sight of the road?

Seeing as, for now anyway, he was locked in, Gregory crossed the hall and opened the door to the estate manager's office. Perhaps if Adam did have something to hide, it was worthwhile him checking.

12

Sunday evenings were meant for relaxation. Why then did Cathy find herself still hunched at her computer, with a stack of ring binders piled high on her desk? It was her own fault really. She should have seen to it long before. If she had kept on top of recording the information as the year had gone on, she might not have been in such a rush at the end.

She had received an email from the general practice appraiser at the end of last week. Cathy knew the woman quite well. She had conducted Cathy's revalidations on two previous occasions. The email had been short and conversational. Just touching base and kicking her up the backside to get her paperwork in order in good time. The woman had said that she would see James also. If Cathy and he could decide on an equally suitable day, she'd do one assessment after the other. James was away, of course, for the following two weeks and Cathy was loath to contact him over the matter. She'd sent the appraiser a quick reply explaining that her senior partner was on annual leave and that they would be in touch soon. It gave her a little breathing space, but not much.

Forms one and two had taken minutes. Merely a quick

reflection on her background and job description. To be honest, she simply cut and pasted from last year's, only needing to amend a few details. The more arduous task was going to be the third part. For this, she was obliged to reflect on her professional development over the year and to provide written detail to back it up. This might involve considering a significant event that had occurred within the practice or a complaint she, or the practice as a whole, had received. Cathy wasn't sure she wanted to do this, so she had decided instead, to do a questionnaire. This, the form stated, should be either sent to her colleagues within the practice, or a randomly selected group of her patients. Within this, they would be asked to rate her effectiveness in communication, her empathy, her skill in working within a team and in involving the patient in creating their own treatment plan.

Cathy groaned. The back of the swivel chair in her small office at home creaked as she stretched. She was getting a headache. It was sitting staring at a computer screen that did it. Having saved what she had done so far, she got up. Her shoulders were stiff and she circled them, hearing the click of the ball and socket joint rotating against tense fascia.

When she had decided to become a general practitioner, she had never imagined that so much of her time would be consumed by paperwork. Of course, there were the usual things; letters to be written for patients, referrals, insurance forms and prescriptions. But over the years, the amount of evidence required to validate her ability to practise had increased exponentially. Clearly, there were some positives to this. Patients could be reassured that they might receive the best care from a clinician, who was now assessed by the health board yearly. This made keeping up to date with medical advances a priority. That had to be a good thing. But if only there wasn't so much to document as proof.

Cathy crossed the room again and looked down at the

computer screen. Her own health was still to be scrutinized. The medical report from her psychiatrist and GP would be attached later. Cathy wouldn't have minded so much if it wasn't for that. And then, she was still to complete the last section of the forms. It was ominously titled: 'Maintaining Trust.' Cathy shook her head and decided that she was in no mood to tackle it just now. She'd come back when she was in a better frame of mind.

Taking her empty coffee cup, she went to the kitchen to make herself something to eat. She'd lost track of time and it was gone six. Outside, it was getting dark already. Her house was on the outskirts of Glainkirk. She was content where she was in many ways. The street was a dead-end so it meant that its residents weren't bothered by through-traffic. Cathy hadn't spoken to her neighbours for weeks. They were all patients at the practice and sometimes she wondered if they avoided her, perhaps out of respect, but also conceivably out of embarrassment. Cathy wished she could tell them that she rarely managed to remember a face or a name, let alone what the person had come in with, she saw so many people over the course of a week. Her regulars, of course, she knew intimately. The people who had unfortunately made it onto the palliative care register; they and their families, she had to become well-acquainted with and sometimes very fast depending on how severe their condition.

Cathy found herself stirring the pot of tinned soup on the stove and thinking of one of her patients, a lovely woman in her mid-fifties who would be lucky to see the end of the month. Cancer could be incredibly cruel. She'd need to go and visit the woman tomorrow. She hoped that she'd had a comfortable weekend. The out-of-hours doctors would have attended to any issues. Cathy had emailed them on Friday afternoon before heading home, to alert them to the lady's deteriorating state. The steam from the soup now rose to her nostrils filling them with the tomatoey aroma. She dispensed the hot liquid and cradled the steaming bowl, yelping as the porcelain burned at her hands. She'd sit through in the living room. It was warmest in there.

She watched the news, kneeling at the coffee table, blowing on the soup, her eyes streaming from taking the first blistering sip. Cathy reflected on her weekend. She'd not been out of the house at all, other than to stock up the cupboards for the week.

Impulsively, she snatched up her mobile phone and searched for the number.

'Well?' came the irritable reply.

Cathy laughed. 'Bad time, is it?'

'Never, but I am annoyed with you.'

'Oh?' Cathy asked, knowing only too well why.

She heard a grunt from the end of the line and then her friend spoke. 'Well?' the other doctor asked. 'Explain yourself. How long has it been? And I have left messages. Don't pretend you haven't got them.'

Cathy laughed again. 'You sound like my bloody mother.'

Suzalinna tutted. 'So, what's new? Why have you been off the radar for so long?'

'James is off on annual leave and it's just me running the show.' She sighed. 'Sorry. I've been trying to sort out my revalidation nonsense today too and the paperwork has been unbelievable.'

Cathy heard her friend snort. 'All reasonable excuses, but none of them cut it. You could have been dead in a ditch for all I knew.'

'Well, you're not far off the truth as it happens.'

Cathy told her old medical school friend the story of her minor collision the previous week.

'Jesus,' Suzalinna said. 'You need to be more careful. I don't want you being wheeled into my department any time soon. Really, we're quite busy enough.'

'How is work?' Cathy asked.

Suzalinna laughed. 'Same old, you know how it gets. Brodie's been off sick, so the rota's a one-in-four now. I'm on nights, as it happens.'

'Oh Suzalinna, I am so sorry. Did I wake you?'

'Don't be ridiculous. I've been up for hours. I'll be heading in soon. I've got paperwork too, you know. It isn't just GPs breaking their backs with work. Anyway, when are you coming over? I was hoping you'd be free sometime this week. Nights finish on Tuesday, so I'm good after that. Saj was asking for you too.'

Cathy smiled at the thought of Suzalinna's affable husband, Saj, also a doctor, but undeniably at his wife's beck and call.

'Oh God, I feel bad saying no, Suz, but honestly, this week is going to be chaos at work. I'll be more on top of things in the coming weeks, I'm sure.'

The phone was silent for a moment and then Suzalinna spoke once more, but with a definite change in tone. 'Just a thought, but I'm wondering, what with the mention of revalidation ...'

Cathy didn't answer and her friend spoke again.

'I know what you're like,' she continued. 'You always do it around this time. It happened last year too. You cut yourself off from everyone and go underground.' Her friend laughed. 'You're like a bloody mole!'

Cathy snorted. 'Hardly,' she said. 'Why would I do that?'

'You know very well,' Suzalinna scolded, but Cathy could hear she was smiling. 'Darling, you've nothing to worry about. You're doing fine. I know that, and so does James. He'd have had a word with you already if he had any concerns. So would your psychiatrist. You will get your fitness to practise ticked off, as you always do.'

Cathy laughed, but it didn't sound convincing. She heard her friend sigh.

'You know, this isn't even about the bipolar. It's not about your time off at all. You've always been like this. Back at medical school, you were just the same when it came to exams. You doubt yourself too much. When are you going to believe that you are in the right place, doing the right thing?'

When Cathy hung up, having finally agreed to stay better in touch, she sighed. Of course, her friend had been quite right, but it wasn't that simple.

13

'Can I have a word later?' Gregory asked the following morning as he and Adam stood together, side-by-side at the cattle court.

The estate manager shrugged. 'As long as it isn't that nonsense about premium haylage again, Oi! Had you heard Greg's latest scheme?' he called to one of the younger farmhands nearby.

The boy snorted and grinned to another lad working beside him. They both rolled their eyes and sniggered.

Gregory felt his face burning. Damn cheek it was. Trying to humiliate him in front of his subordinates. His idea had been a valid one too.

Adam was moving off though. 'You crack on with the fence in Potter's Field, there's a good man,' he said.

Patronising bastard, Gregory thought, but he didn't speak and instead, smiled wickedly at the back of Adam's head. Oh, he'd have a word later alright, and then Adam-bloody-Foster would be in no position to ignore him.

That day, Gregory had left the house with a spring in his step. Even Fiona had noticed the change in him.

'Chirpy today, aren't you?' she asked as she prepared to leave the house herself. 'You're usually in a huff on a Monday morning knowing that the lads over the weekend will have been slap-dash.'

Gregory snorted. Right enough he was. The labourers that often covered the weekend rota were lazy. Last week, he had returned to find that one of the cows had delivered and the fools hadn't bothered to tag the calf. Bloody joke it was. Distrusting the young fools, he'd driven past the court last night to check on the cows after leaving the estate office via a window. He wondered if Adam might notice it hadn't been locked when he came in that following morning. An oversight on his part, he'd probably think. Careless of him. Gregory smiled again, thinking about his discovery the previous night. Two finds in a day; the coins and then this.

He had lain awake half the night thinking about how best to proceed with things. It concerned him that Adam, on exiting the office, might have spotted his jeep parked up on the main road, not a hundred yards from the office. Gregory hoped that the estate manager wasn't forewarned. Surprise, he felt was the key to exposing the oily man. There was little doubt that the advantage lay with him, but Gregory knew that Adam was clever. No-one could deny that, and if he was to outwit him, he'd have to go about the thing carefully.

That morning, he had looked across at his wife, thinking of the showdown that lay ahead that day. She had lost her house keys and was scrabbling around in the fruit bowl looking for them.

'I'll be back and forward passing the house today,' he said as he watched her. 'I've got an appointment to get my gun licence signed off late afternoon. We've nothing worth stealing. I'll leave the door open. I never usually lock the damn thing anyway.'

Fiona tutted and continued to search. A smile pricked at

Gregory's lips. Nothing of value currently, but if he was correct about the far side of Potter's Field, he might well have something of worth in a number of weeks. And then, of course, he hadn't even accounted for the potential revenue that might come from his estate manager. His luck had certainly changed, that was for sure.

Fiona had found her keys. She held them aloft and smiled. 'I was thinking about having Rosemary and David over next week,' she said. 'You'd find the time?'

Gregory had rejected this suggestion several times before. He knew that she was choosing her moment to raise the matter again. Let her have her bit of fun, he thought. She'd go off to her silly work thinking she'd outsmarted him. Caught him at a good time to ask.

'Uh-huh,' he said, slipping his arms into his jacket.

His wife's eyes flashed. 'Just an informal thing. I know David wants to have a word with you. He's been desperate to get onto one of the shoots and I suppose he sees you as his ticket. You'd manage to arrange it if he wanted, wouldn't you?'

Gregory shrugged.

'I feel we owe them a favour,' Fiona continued coming towards him. 'Rosemary got me the job in the first place, after all, and then she covered for me on Friday when I was late too. Being friendly makes all the difference, you know?' She touched the lapel on his jacket and patted it. 'A favour for a favour.' She leaned in and he kissed her cheek. 'Anyway, I'll catch you tonight,' she continued, stepping away. 'I'll cook something nice. A roast perhaps. Although, I've never done one before. I'll need to get help from my mum.'

Gregory rolled his eyes and didn't speak. He could think of nothing worse than sitting down for some daft dinner party with Fiona's fancy friends, especially if it involved input from his mother-in-law. But no matter, he had far more important things to think of that day. He'd not allow anything to dampen his mood.

In the end, he didn't find time to get to the estate office until after one, which left him only a short time before his doctor's appointment. All morning, he had been busy with the cattle and then overseeing some of the fencing going up in one of the bottom fields. When he did arrive at the office, Adam was busy. Mr Dewhurst was in speaking to him, and Gregory stood outside by the gun cabinet behind which he had hidden only the day before, listening to the men's voices. He couldn't make out what was being said, but he heard Mr Dewhurst's unrelenting speech, quiet and level, and then Adam's; higher-pitched, persuasive and ingratiating. When the old man left, Gregory stepped forward with a smile, but Mr Dewhurst seemed in a hurry and did not acknowledge him. Gregory tutted. Bloody typical it was. Invisible, that was about right. The cheek. He approached Adam's door and knocked. Although he was quite determined, his hands were clammy and his heart was pounding in his ears.

'Yes?' came the estate manager's voice.

Gregory opened the door.

'Greg. Really? I'm up to my eyeballs in work. Can't you look after things yourself for once in your life and leave me to do my job in peace?'

Gregory swallowed and shifted his feet.

'Well?' Adam said. 'I've got a hundred and one things to see to today. You are very much at the bottom of my list. If it's not important, piss off. I've had it up to here with bloody labourers for one day.'

Gregory took a deep breath and came fully into the room. He closed the door behind him.

Adam, who had obviously thought he had dismissed him, looked up in annoyance. 'Well then? What's this all about? I told you I'm busy.' he repeated.

'It won't take long,' Gregory said. His voice was calm and the tone hinted at a smile, although none came to his lips 'I wanted a quiet word about my position again, Adam.'

The other man looked at him in disbelief but before he could speak, Gregory went on. 'I've just seen Mr Dewhurst leaving. I can run after him and have a quick word if you're too busy, but I'd like that promotion I'd mentioned to you before, Adam. That's why I've come. And I'd like a significant raise in my salary too. That's if it's not too much trouble.'

14

Cathy re-read the form and looked up. The man's face was ruddy. He wore dusty jeans and a heavy, checkered jacket. He ran the palm of a hand across his face; the stubble sounded like sandpaper.

'Nothing's changed,' he said as if in answer to a question and then laughed.

She returned her attention to the notes, checking for details of the last time he had been in to consult someone.

'Just more paperwork to waste your time with,' he continued. 'I wanted to come in and hurry it along. The police said they'd sent it to you a while ago. I need it, you see? They did the house check a few weeks back. It's all in order.' He paused and then his face lit up. 'Hey, didn't I give you a pull out of a ditch the other week? I did! I was on the way back from taking a load of fence-posts down to the bottom field. I was sure I recognised your face.'

Cathy smiled. 'Well, yes. It was you, was it? I was in such a fluster, I'm afraid I didn't notice your face even. Thank you once again for that.'

The man nodded. 'Tractor comes in handy. You're not the first. Everyone takes that bend too fast.'

Cathy was going to explain that speed hadn't been the issue, but rather it had been her soft-hearted attempt to avoid a pheasant that had done the damage. She thought better of it and nodded instead.

'I understand you've held the licence for some time. Can you tell me roughly how long?'

The man leaned back in his seat. 'Oh, years and years,' he said. 'They get updated every five, I think.' He sounded as if he was going to yawn. 'The last time, some old boy signed the thing. Dr Longmuir, was it? I don't come in often; you'll see that in my notes.' He grinned. 'Much damage to the car then?'

Cathy turned and looked at the computer screen. 'No damage, thank you.' She quickly scanned the records for relevant information. The man was indeed an infrequent attender. He'd last been in to see Linda, their salaried doctor, a year and a half ago. It had been about a chest infection.

'Just a few questions. Can I ask about your mood?' Cathy began.

The man snorted and raised his hands above his head in a stretch. 'No bother there,' he said, resting his linked fingers behind his head.

Cathy looked once more at the computer.

'I don't see what the issue is,' he continued. 'Honestly, nothing's changed at all. Your colleague signed it right away the last time. He didn't ask a thing.'

Cathy doubted if this was true, knowing James to be meticulous in his work. She looked up. 'I'm just doing my job,' she said pleasantly. 'I know it's a bit of a bore but I'm treating you no differently to anyone else I might see for a gun licence renewal.' Cathy smiled again, trying to find some common ground. 'Can you tell me a little about your work? What is it you do?' she asked.

The man puffed his cheeks out and then exhaled in annoyance. 'Farm work. Obviously. You know that already. You saw me in the tractor.' He then gestured to his clothes. 'I see to the cattle; I sort the fencing. It's rough, it's outside and I enjoy it. And before you ask, no there are no problems with my mind. I'm not planning on blowing my brains out any time soon.'

Cathy blinked slowly. The questions she was asking weren't so unusual or offensive. 'Tell me,' she continued, her voice not displaying her wonder at the man's attitude towards her. 'How often are you required to use the gun?'

'Daily if I want to. It's not a requirement, as you put it, but it keeps the pests down. We supervise proper shoots but don't often take part. It's too busy for that. I check that other people are holding their guns properly. That shows you how skilled I am. I've been shooting since I was a kid. Used to practise with my old man's gun to shoot the rabbits when I was still at primary school.'

Cathy looked up, suddenly making the connection. She experienced a dreadful sinking feeling. She hadn't realised, but of course, *that* was who he was. She was speaking with Fiona Warrender's husband. The girl had only been in last week. Why hadn't she known when she called him into her room? She should have remembered the name. Cathy recalled the young woman's startled look and the bruise on her wrist. And here in front of her now, was the very man that Cathy suspected of possibly mistreating her.

It was quite a dilemma. Cathy sat still, trying to think. Of course, if the man had no mental health issues other than a dubious attitude, she could hardly refuse to grant him her signature. She would be following the guidelines scrupulously. But then, with this extra knowledge of his ill-temper at home and admittedly, without confirmation, her supposition that he might be behaving abusively towards his wife, what should she do? She had no substantiated reason to believe that he might use the weapon on himself, or anyone else. If she was filling out the form properly, she would state this alone and could do so with a clear conscience.

The man was getting more restless. He shifted in his seat and then began to drum his grubby fingernails on the desk.

If James had been there, sitting next-door consulting along-side her, he would have been delighted to advise. His counsel would have been pragmatic and considered. He would have known from years of experience what to do. But James wasn't there. She was the only doctor consulting that afternoon.

'Well?' the man said.

Cathy suddenly felt both hot and dizzy. Making an impulsive judgement, she got up. She held onto the edge of her desk to steady herself. 'I'm afraid I can't sign the form now without looking over your notes more thoroughly,' she said.

The man set his jaw and a wave of blotchy red crept from his neck to his cheeks. 'Excuse me?' he asked quietly.

'I understand it's not how things have been done in the past, but the guidelines for general practitioners have changed some-what in the last five years. I doubt there'll be a problem. Your licence doesn't run out until the following month anyway and I'm sure we'll have things in order well before then.'

'Look,' he said, his voice suddenly disarming. 'I can see you maybe don't do many of these things.' He waved towards the form. 'I don't expect you to like guns. But they're a necessity in my line of work. We do it all officially. We fill out all the paper-work on time, we even pay for the privilege. Your signature doesn't come cheap, Doctor. I've taken half the afternoon off work. Left the calving to some school-leaver to come to you. I didn't think it would be this difficult.'

Cathy hesitated and he continued.

'I can promise you; my gun is kept secure and safe. I am the only person handling it. When I use it, it is to kill rabbits or to shoot pheasants on the estate. The estate itself is run to a very high standard. It has to be. We have visitors coming to us, paying hundreds of pounds to shoot. Bloodsports aren't everyone's cup of tea. Not mine, if I'm honest, but it's what I know. It's my background. Please don't discriminate because of your ethical beliefs.'

He had misunderstood her reasoning, and it was probably just as well. Cathy wavered, her heart now thudding in her ears.

'I don't know what else I can say,' the man continued. 'I thought, having dragged you out of a ditch the other week, it might make you more agreeable.'

She looked at the man's face. He smiled back at her.

She wanted this to end. Reaching for her pen, she signed. When she looked up, he looked triumphant.

'Thanks, Doc,' he said. 'You'll not regret it.'

When he left, she sat motionless for some time. Cathy hoped with all her heart that he was right. But all that afternoon, her thoughts returned to Mr Warrender's young wife, her frightened eyes and the bruise on her wrist. Why had she signed the form?

15

'Well, I hope there's been no more talk of poison if we're being invited to the house?'

Rosemary cast her husband a disparaging look. 'Don't be ludicrous. That was Fiona exaggerating as usual. From what she said this week, he's been in fine spirits and the marriage is back on track. All that silly talk of him trying to kill her was juvenile nonsense. She is younger than us, remember?'

'Only by a few years,' David said. 'I thought the last of it was that her head was aching every time he made her anything to drink, and her hair was falling out.' He looked at his wife from over the local newspaper and grinned.

Rosemary crossed the room and perched on the arm of the chair. 'Don't you want to come then? I thought you'd be pleased. You've been going on about getting in with Mr Dewhurst for months. Gregory might get you onto a shoot. But please don't start by trying to wangle an invite up to the big house.'

'Through their cattleman? I hardly think so, Rose. You know that as well as I do.' He shuffled the paper, adjusting the pages so that they were in line. 'Gregory won't pull much weight. I need to speak to that estate man, Adam, without stirring too much notice. He's the fellow. He'll know the lay of the land before I go crashing in and making a fool of myself. Is that what your friend promised then? A ticket to a shoot? Seems a bit desperate, no?'

'Desperate for what? Our company? I hate it when you talk like that. Don't be such a bloody snob. From what I hear, Gregory is far more than a simple labourer. Fiona said he's been promoted. And what if that was all he did? What then? I only work as a personal assistant. Does that make me inferior too?'

David deliberately closed his paper and folded the pages over. He placed the newsprint on the occasional table in front of him and met his wife's gaze steadily. 'Undoubtedly inferior,' he answered. 'I've already offered you a job at my office, but you're too proud. I suppose I can bring the brochures though. I doubt there's much point. That girl Fiona's got her head in the clouds. They'll not buy one of the new builds from us. Too upmarket for the likes of them.'

Although she knew he was being sardonic, Rosemary was in no mood for his negativity. She got up abruptly, smoothing down the folds in her skirt. 'Well, I've said yes to Fiona already anyway, so it's too late to back out now. I'll iron your pink shirt. The one with the holes for the cufflinks.'

'You're too efficient,' he said. 'Sort every bloody thing.'

THREE DAYS LATER, they stood on the doorstep to Fiona and Gregory's cottage. David had driven and agreed that he'd only have one drink. Rosemary clasped a bottle of wine. 'Wasted on them,' her husband had said in the car. 'Why you couldn't have grabbed a cheaper one, I don't know.' Rosemary had ignored his griping and wondered aloud if they should stop also at the petrol station on the way to pick up a bunch of flowers.

'For goodness sake, behave,' she said to her husband as they now waited. From inside, a female voice could be heard repeatedly calling Gregory's name. 'If you've nothing nice to say ...' Rosemary continued, but the door was opened and Fiona, red-cheeked and flustered, stood before them. She was wearing a blue cotton dress and over this, a striped apron, which was heavily stained.

'Christ alone knows where he is!' Fiona said. 'Must have nipped out without me realising when I was in the shower. Hello David, nice to see you again.' She turned to Rosemary. 'Jesus, Rosemary. Thank God you're here. You'd better give me a hand. The gravy's gone to pot and my mum's not a been a bit of help today.'

Stepping inside, Rosemary kissed her friend on the cheek and passed her the bottle of wine.

Fiona moving back through the house, abandoned the wine on the kitchen table. Her hands fluttered in agitation and as she turned, she knocked her hip on the edge of the counter and cursed. The smell of cooking hung heavily in the air. Rosemary watched her husband glancing around disdainfully before hanging his overcoat on the stair bannister. She followed Fiona through, only half-listening to her friend's nervous chatter about how useless Gregory had been that day by not helping her get the place tidy, and how unfair it had been of her mother to choose that very day to head up to Forkieth with her sister on a shopping trip.

'I'd told her she was meant to be on standby,' Fiona was saying, 'but she'd made up her mind. You'll not mind if it's a bit rough around the edges though, will you David?' Fiona said, looking over Rosemary's shoulder.

Rosemary didn't dare turn to see her husband's expression but instead crossed the kitchen and began opening cupboard doors. 'Wine glasses?' she asked.

'Oh, over in that one,' Fiona said, glancing to the cupboard in despair. 'Help yourselves. Gregory has Port somewhere and there's beer in the cupboard below the stairs. We should've put some in the fridge for you. David, had you wanted a beer? I'm so sorry. What a bloody mess it all is.'

David still stood in the kitchen doorway. 'I'll make do with whatever,' he said, 'Don't suppose you've any sloe gin?' Rosemary shot him a look and he smiled roguishly at her.

Poor Fiona wiped her hands on her apron. Rosemary thought that the girl looked close to tears. 'No, I don't suppose we do,' she said. 'They drink it before the shoots, don't they? That and the port, but Gregory's not fond of the stuff. I could get him to go out, David, when he comes back. He'd get some from the estate office probably, if you'd like. I'm sure it wouldn't be a bother. We could replace it on Monday. They've got a shoot this weekend so the office will be open until late tonight. I think Adam likes to get all the paperwork sorted beforehand. Some of them won't have their own guns, so he'll be organising the estate's ones ready, along with the documentation, I suppose.'

'Ignore David, he's driving so he'll just have water,' Rosemary said as Fiona began opening drawers apparently at random. 'So, the manager-chap and Gregory are getting on better then?' Rosemary asked, crossing the room with a glass of water before passing it to her husband. 'Go through to the living room and leave us to talk,' she said severely.

'We're eating through there too,' Fiona called after David's retreating figure. 'I hope you're not fussed, Rosemary. I set up the fold-out table there. You know we don't have a dining room. But David won't mind, will he? David!' she called. 'Would you grab a couple of beers from under the stairs? I'll put them in the fridge now or Gregory'll say I've forgotten that too.'

David seemed to be out of earshot, so Rosemary instead fetched four bottles from under the stairs and rearranged things in the fridge so that they fitted. She then poured a glass of wine for her friend and told her that it would all be perfect. 'So, Gregory's no longer trying to poison you?' she teased.

Fiona grinned. 'I promise you'll be safe eating here tonight. All of this has been my doing.'

'And he seems happier at work?' Rosemary asked, beginning to lift the lids on the pots that sat on the hob. 'You know we could have had a takeaway, Fiona, this is such a lot of trouble you've gone to.'

Fiona smiled. 'It's funny about his work as you say. Strangely, I'd never have suggested going for a bottle from the office before. Quite frosty it used to be and asking a favour would have been out of the question. But this week, there's been a bit of a change. Obviously, I told you about the promotion. Adam, that's the estate manager, seems to have mellowed. He even came past the house for a word with Greg the other night. Chummy as anything. I heard Gregory laughing his head off on the doorstep. I told him he should've invited Adam in for a drink after he'd gone but you know what Greg's like. Not good at social stuff at all.'

'David's just the same,' Rosemary said.

Fiona smiled but didn't look convinced. 'No idea what happened to smooth things over,' Fiona went on. 'Greg said that he and Adam had finally come to an understanding, but I haven't a clue what that means. Oh, but he can tell you himself.' The front door banged. 'And where have you been?' Fiona asked as Gregory appeared in the kitchen.

'I told you,' he said. 'Cattle.' He looked at the kitchen table, where David had left the estate agents' brochure for the new builds up in Glainkirk town centre. His face twisted in disgust.

Rosemary looked from Gregory to Fiona. She had thought that things were a good deal better between the two, but it seemed that Gregory was in no mood to be shown up by his wife, and certainly not in his own house.

'They've been here for nearly half an hour,' Fiona said, scowling.

'Hardly that. Just ten minutes. How are things, Gregory? Nice to see you,' Rosemary said smoothly. 'Work keeping you busy then?'

Gregory looked at her but didn't answer. 'I'm going up for a shower,' he said and turned.

Fiona swore and banged down the pan she had been holding. The boiling water slopped up over the edge and she jumped back.

'Calm down,' Rosemary told her. 'Let's get things dished up and ready. We'll do it together.'

The meal itself wasn't a great success. Fiona, clearly unpractised in such matters, had produced something that was at least edible but not especially enjoyable. Rosemary did her best to accommodate her friend, talking animatedly at times about their experiences at work. Rosemary was disappointed to see that Gregory made little effort to make his wife feel relaxed. Admittedly, David wasn't playing ball either. He had been pushing the same slimy roast potato around his plate for a good five minutes. Both men looked as if they would rather be anywhere else. David, she knew wanted to get home to watch the football and Gregory, she assumed, was yearning to be with his beloved cows. She asked him about his work a couple of times.

'Set to change,' he said and she raised her eyebrows. 'Oh yes.' Gregory laughed.

Rosemary had noticed him emptying the rest of the bottle of wine they had brought into his glass. She doubted he was usually a wine drinker at all.

'Yes. Big changes are afoot,' he scoffed, his face a deep, mottled-red.

'In what way?' David asked, finally laying his fork and knife down. 'I had heard that old Dewhurst was in some financial difficulty. There's been talk of the house being opened up for weddings it's so desperate. You'd think he'd want to sell off some of the land. Worth a fair price to a property developer.'

Gregory snorted loudly and Rosemary saw Fiona shifting in her seat.

'Mr Dewhurst,' Gregory said in a mocking tone. 'The man doesn't have a clue what's under his bloody nose. He might be in less financial trouble if he listened to me.'

'Gregory, what on earth ...?'

He turned to his wife. 'You laugh at my metal-detecting, but what if I'd found something? What if it was more than anyone imagined? What then?'

'Don't be ridiculous,' Fiona said and shot Rosemary a desperate look.

'Anyway,' Rosemary said. 'Let's hope that Mr Dewhurst manages to save the situation. Such a beautiful, old house when you look up that way from the road.'

Gregory sneered. 'Old man doesn't know what's going on. Certainly, doesn't know what his staff are doing.' The farmhand took another swig from his glass. 'About time the damn fool opened his eyes, but I'll not be the one to say anything. Not unless I have to.'

'Fiona said that there was a shoot planned for the week-end?' David asked, choosing to ignore his comments. 'I heard that they were charging three hundred a day. Seems odd that the estate's in difficulty given that he's doing well commercially. I suppose the house must be a nightmare to maintain. And there are the wages to pay. How many staff does he have now?'

Gregory seemed to have lost interest and Fiona answered for him. 'I'm not sure, David. I think as far as the farm side of things goes, they must have ten or twelve, but goodness knows about the house as you say. Mr Dewhurst has others too, the gamekeeper ...'

Gregory's face turned purple and he grunted loudly.

'David's only asking because he's been dying to go on a shoot for years but he's never found a route in,' Rosemary said hurriedly.

David frowned. 'I'll not deny it. We've had a pop at clay pigeons in the past, haven't we Rose? I was pretty good ...'

Gregory guffawed and slapped the table with the palm of his hand. 'Clays? You have to be kidding me. Clays? It's nothing like a real shoot. Clays,' he mocked, shaking his head in disgust.

'David's not from a farming background, I suppose,' Rosemary said quickly, knowing only too well that her husband would be furious. She glanced across at him. He glared back.

But Gregory seemed not to notice and was still chuckling to himself. 'Clays,' he kept saying again and again.

'You'd get David on a shoot, wouldn't you Greg?' Fiona asked, her eyes imploring.

'You want in on a shoot?' Gregory eventually asked, mopping the imaginary tears from his eyes. 'You really want in on a shoot? I can get you on one tomorrow. Easy. I'm in with the gaffer and he'll not say no if I ask.'

Rosemary looked at her husband. It was clear that he was going through a range of emotions. Knowing him only too well, Rosemary recognized that although it might dent his pride to accept the offer, if he did not, he would forever kick himself.

'Alright then,' David finally said, lifting a glass of water from the table. 'That'd be fine.'

'Christ alone knows why you want to,' Gregory went on. 'Bloody awful sport. No skill in it; taking a pop at those fat, feckless birds. Bred to die. Nurtured from the hand by your pal.' He spat this comment at his wife, who seemed to recoil in her seat. 'Bloody graceless creatures,' he continued sneeringly, turning back to David and Rosemary. 'They don't stand a bloody chance. Not like rabbiting,' he continued. 'At least that has a purpose. Pests they are. Destroy the crops. You're so into your hunting, I'll let you have a pop at a few tonight if you want. Hundreds of them behind the house. My gun's under the stairs.' Gregory began pushing his chair back, but it was clear that he had had far too much to drink and he swayed and clutched at the table.

'Sit down, idiot,' Fiona hissed, but he righted himself and stormed from the room leaving everyone dumbfounded and embarrassed.

Following the meal, Gregory and David ended up talking about guns and goodness knows what else on the back doorstep, leaving the two women to clear up. Tempers had abated thank goodness but Rosemary was glad when the evening came to an end and they could leave the stilted conversation and fragile atmosphere.

'Honestly, I can't thank you enough for having us,' she said to her friend as she said goodbye. 'It's our turn next time.'

Fiona kissed her on the cheek, her lips cool and dry on Rosemary's skin.

'If this shoot thing comes to anything tomorrow, why don't I come over as well? It might be fun. We'll make a picnic for the boys and take them their lunch after the first drive,' Rosemary suggested.

'Oh, please, Rosemary. Yes. Do come.'

Rosemary was surprised, and Fiona must have seen it in her face.

'Please,' she said again. Her eyes were wide and Rosemary was sure that a message was implied behind the look.

She wanted to ask Fiona if everything was really alright between her and Gregory, but then, David appeared in the doorway with his jacket, laughing. It seemed that the awkwardness from earlier was now forgotten.

'Come on,' he said. 'That's enough girly gossip for one night.'

As they drove home in silence, Rosemary wondered why her friend had been so insistent that she return the following day. Had the expression Fiona had given her, been one of fear? Rosemary had a horrible sense of unease about the thing. Oddly, she recalled once more the words of the old woman on the train. 'Resentment can be dangerous,' she had said. Was she right after all? Was Fiona in danger? Rosemary thought of Gregory's gun beneath the stairs and hoped with all her heart that she was wrong.

16

Cathy arrived home late to find that James had left a message on her answer machine. He sounded relaxed and she wondered if he'd had a drink before he called. Perhaps the time off work was just what he needed? These past few months had undoubtedly been a strain on the practice and being senior partner, James had borne the brunt of it.

Dropping her car keys on the hall table, she listened to James's message for the second time. All he was saying was that he was there for her if she needed him. She knew that he meant this quite genuinely, but she also knew that she would rather do anything than phone him while he was on a well-deserved break from work.

Cathy kicked off her ankle boots by the front door and went through to the kitchen in her stockinged feet. The floor was icy cold and she winced.

Her thoughts once more returned to the awkward consultation the previous week and she wondered why it still played on her mind. Had she been overreacting in the first place, in thinking that Fiona Warrender was in danger? If she hadn't met the young woman's husband since, she might well have forgotten about the whole thing by now and put it down to her overactive imagination. But she had met Gregory Warrender, and had instinctively disliked him, even without linking the two consultations.

Cathy shook her head. It wasn't like her. Usually, she hoped she was impartial and fair to everyone who came into her surgery. She recalled the man's consultation and his sly way of dropping into the conversation their previous meeting. At the time, she had been so eager to get him out of the room that she had allowed herself to be manipulated. Cathy crossed the kitchen, shaking her head ruefully. She had done something she had intuitively felt was wrong. Odd to have been swayed so easily. Over the years, she had kicked enough drug-seekers out of her room. She had been shouted at, even spat at a couple of times. Why then, had Gregory Warrender been so different?

Opening the fridge, she removed the chilled bottle of white wine. She wasn't in the habit of drinking these days having been warned off the stuff by her psychiatrist. Still, she poured the yellow-clear liquid into her glass and slouched against the countertop, enjoying her first sip. Why had she signed the gun licence form? She had been halfway to the door, ready to kick Gregory out. She had already told him her reason for not signing the damn thing. What on earth had caused her to change her mind – to sit down, to take the pen and sign? Cathy swirled the wine around the glass. She didn't know why she had done it, but she prayed that she'd not live to regret it.

That evening, she was in no humour to return to her revalidation paperwork. Instead, she sat in silence, watching the pictures on the television, but not listening to what was said. When it came to ten o'clock, she found that she had drunk almost three-quarters of the bottle. She got up unsteadily. Her friend Suzalinna would be furious if she knew. She had repeatedly chastised Cathy in the past for not looking after herself.

When she finally lay in bed hoping for the emptiness to swallow her, she instead saw Gregory Warrender's mottled face, and on it was a look of triumph.

17

'Didn't you hear me last night?' Fiona asked.

Gregory had just come in and was removing his muddy boots at the front door. He grunted. The truth was, he'd slept like the dead. Something dodgy in the wine, he thought. That morning, he woke to a pounding headache and sick stomach It didn't help that he'd agreed to the shoot that day. God alone knew how Adam had persuaded him. He'd said that Mr Dewhurst would be there though, which was a rarity given that the old man was getting on. A few VIPs might be coming too. Now that they had an understanding, Gregory could see that Adam might well continue to put good things in his path. The VIPs tipped astronomically well if a shoot was successful. Gregory understood that the estate had an arrangement so that all tips were collected together and split equally amongst the beaters, but he supposed that Adam would be in no position to argue if he asked for a greater cut this time.

'I was up three times,' Fiona was saying.

Gregory turned and observed his wife for the first time that morning. She looked haggard.

'God, I hope Rosemary and David weren't the same. How embarrassing if I've managed to poison us all,' she said.

Gregory snorted and moved through to the kitchen. 'You seem obsessed with poison at the moment,' he said and began washing his hands in the sink. Fiona had flung open the windows allowing the greasy smell of bacon to escape the confines of the room. He shook his hands and then dried them on a tea towel, something he knew irritated his wife.

'What time are you starting?' she asked. 'Help yourself, I don't have the stomach for it.' She pushed the dish with bacon across the countertop. 'Toast's just done too.'

Gregory wasn't feeling up to breakfast either, but knowing he had a long day ahead, he took a plate all the same and made himself an oily sandwich.

'Ten,' he said. 'But we'll not be doing the first drive until eleven-thirty by the time they faff around.'

'Is David coming here first then?'

He shook his head but didn't speak. He supposed that David would be going straight up to the estate office. He had still to check with Adam about adding him onto the shoot that day, but he assumed there wouldn't be a problem.

Gregory finished his toast and wiped the crumbs from his overalls onto the floor.

'You're changing I assume? I laid the jacket out already. Are you just beating today, or shooting too?'

Gregory slid his plate into the sink, which Fiona had just filled with fresh soapy water.

'I'll be back after seven,' he said, ignoring his wife's question before he left the room. He heard Fiona tutting and then she followed him to the bottom of the stairs.

'We're coming though, me and Rosemary. We'll be there at lunchtime. She's coming here and we're making a picnic together. Were you so drunk last night that you don't remember?

I couldn't believe it when you started going on about those bloody bits of metal you'd found. Do you even remember that? David was trying not to yawn at one point.'

He grunted and continued up the stairs. He couldn't be doing with Fiona's nonsense today. He wished she wasn't coming, and certainly not with her fancy friend Rosemary. Gregory had seen the way the pair of them had looked at him across the table last night.

But things weren't so bad really, he reminded himself. Gregory had already considered that as David was obviously a complete novice, he'd be unlikely to be in the same group. David would be assigned a set of toffs who'd need a step-by-step briefing on how to hold a bloody gun before they headed out. Adam would do that. He always did so that the insurance was in order. He'd be even more particular if Mr Dewhurst was standing over him watching.

Gregory would have to check his own gun, come to think of it. It was a while since he'd had it properly out of the case. Last night he had shown it to David while the girls had been tidying up. The foolish man hadn't a clue. There was no way Gregory would have allowed him to touch the thing. He wondered how Adam would coach the idiot that day. Of course, Adam, if he was being pedantic, would need the paperwork for his gun as well as the rest. Gregory wondered where he had left it after having the thing signed off by the silly woman GP. Probably in the kitchen drawer. That was where most things ended up. Fiona would undoubtedly know but he'd not ask.

As he pulled the front door to, having located his gun's paperwork, not in the kitchen drawer but actually in his gun case under the stairs, Gregory called goodbye to his wife and left. He drove swiftly to the estate office, keen to have a word with Adam before anyone else arrived. Gregory considered that the role of blackmailer had not come easily to him.

Despite his power over Adam, he still caught himself momentarily questioning if what he was doing was right. But as he turned the car on the gravelled area in front of the office and saw Adam's polished Audi parked at a jaunty angle, he set his jaw firmly. No, Adam's luck had run out. Gregory recalled the years of subservience at the other man's hands, his way of talking down to him. His lack of interest in anyone other than himself.

Gregory got out and slammed the door to his jeep. No, when he had walked into the room that fateful afternoon and seen what Adam had been up to, that had been his defining moment. He'd not miss this opportunity.

THEY SET out after eleven following Adam's preliminary talk on shooting etiquette. Gregory stood at the side by the gun cabinets. They had been unlocked already and all the participants who were borrowing a gun from the estate would be assigned theirs for the day when Adam was finished. The more seasoned shooters always brought their own. Gregory had already noticed one of the so-called VIPs handling an expensive-looking model. He preferred the over-under style of gun himself. The pumps that Adam lent out were bloody awful. Granted, for the less experienced shot, they were lighter, and admittedly, they gave the novice an extra go rather than the two shots the other gun afforded, but there was no comparison.

Mr Dewhurst was still to arrive. No doubt he'd swan in just as the drinks were being handed out, a ridiculous tradition, given that they were all about to head out with dangerous weapons. He nodded at David who was hovering uncertainly by the door. The man was clearly out of his comfort zone and this pleased Gregory indescribably. Adam hadn't questioned Gregory's declaration that he had invited an extra for the shoot, but then Adam was in no position to argue.

'I knew it wouldn't be a bother,' Gregory had smirked earlier, watching the other man's face redden.

'This time we have space,' Adam had conceded.

'This time? Any time.' Gregory had asserted. 'I don't suppose you'd argue now, would you? Even if I turned up with ten add-ons for a shoot, you'd agree.'

Adam had turned on his heel and busied himself with the paperwork.

A slow smile spread across Gregory's face in recollection. Bloody Adam Foster.

When Adam's little pantomime of explaining the shoot protocol was done with, Gregory, along with three more experienced men, drove ahead. He had been correct in his assumption that David would be at a different peg. Once in position, he watched as the other Land Rovers pulled up to the field beside theirs. They'd take the first marker, he told Adam. His job was to oversee the men on either side of him. He would, of course, have an opportunity to shoot too, if they proved competent. Despite their protestations of skill, only by the second drive would he be sure. To be honest, Gregory didn't much care. He'd killed more birds and rabbits before he'd left school than most of these men would do in a lifetime. For now, he left his gun in the back of the truck. David was at the far side of the field with Adam. He watched as Adam went through the explanation of how to correctly load the gun again. Gregory snorted. Damn joke it was.

Gregory didn't join in with the chatter at his peg. The toffs were playing at being great sports, joshing one another and asking if there was a prize for the greatest number of pheasants that day. The beaters, in contrast, stood forlornly at the side with their dogs, looking cold. Gregory had already seen Adam's two spaniels in the back of his truck and he supposed that if Adam himself wasn't shooting, he'd get his dogs to pick up.

Mr Dewhurst, having failed to materialise at the estate office, then arrived. Gregory watched the old man peering this way and that, and then, on spotting Adam, he made a beeline for him. The two stood taking for some time. Gregory was growing impatient. It was nearly eleven-thirty now and they'd not even started. What the hell was Adam thinking?

When they were finally given the shout, the beaters got to work. Waving their flags, they sent the dogs plunging into the undergrowth. It took a moment or two and Gregory wondered if they'd chosen a bad first drive, but then came the barrage of indignant shrieks and the inevitable flapping of brown feathers. The female birds were more reticent, their dull, mottled coffees only visible after the russet and green of the males. There would usually be a shout from Adam to signal the start, but someone further down the line had begun. And then, they all followed. The volley of shots was deafening. Despite only lasting less than a minute, the echoing booms seemed to go on forever. He had watched the men beside him as they shot, keen to assess their skill. A determined look of concentration on one man's face as he took down two, the frustrated absorption of another as he missed, only managing to catch a bird's flailing wing. The smell of smoke and gunpowder hung heavy in the air. Gregory, despite being a seasoned shot himself, felt the saliva pool in his mouth as a wave of nausea crashed over him.

The dogs were sent in to collect. Adam Foster's spaniel dived into the undergrowth and returned with one, a large male pheasant. The bird was too big for the dog to carry and its body hung slack and bloody, trailing horribly between the dog's front legs. The mound of birds before Adam grew and the shooters laughed and congratulated one another on their spoils. Few of the birds would go home. That was the waste of the exercise.

Maybe one or two would be stuffed into some novice's freezer, a trophy to impress their wife with. The rest would be dumped. Reared by hand from poults by Adam Foster's flunky, Kenneth. Tended to and nurtured daily by the dreadful man. Any potential predators would have been trapped or shot by the gamekeeper. All simply to satisfy the bloodthirst of these arrogant fools.

18

By lunchtime, Gregory's nausea had not subsided. He stood by the Land Rover, barely hearing the senseless chatter around him. He saw nearby that David seemed to have established a mateyness with Adam which was repulsive to the extreme. Not just this, but to Gregory's absolute disgust, he'd even seen Kenneth the damn gamekeeper arriving and joining in in the jovialities.

The group had already driven to the next position in preparation for the afternoon's shooting. It was a well-used spot, across from Potter's Field where Gregory had been only the weekend before. The river that ran parallel to the woodland was high following rain over the past few days. It was from here that they often beat, allowing the shooters to aim across the water.

Gregory cast his gaze beyond the woodland, towards the spot where he had done his careful excavating. Despite his low mood, Gregory roused himself, thinking of the treasure that might lie beneath their very feet. How amusing it was to know this, while Mr Dewhurst strutted around acting like the lord of the manor, even though most of the party must surely have heard how dire the man's finances were.

Adam had said that the second drive would begin at two. The beaters, along with some of the house staff, had brought flasks of hot drinks and soup. Small groups of raucous gentries stood by or leaned on, the cars. Someone was calling out for a shot of something stronger to warm the cockles. Gregory grimaced in revulsion.

'Well, I thought you'd be in a better mood by now. I heard it was a successful morning.'

Gregory swivelled and saw his wife. Over her shoulder, he noted Rosemary approaching her husband too.

'Oh?' he asked. 'And who told you that? Lover-boy, Kenneth?'

'Oh, for Christ sake, don't,' Fiona hissed, glancing around them.

'I don't care who hears,' he said coolly.

'What is it with you?' she asked. 'We came with lunch.'

'You needn't have bothered. I'm not hungry. Go and chat with your fancy friends.' Gregory began to move away.

'Gregory ...'

He went to the back of the Land Rover and ignoring his wife, began to unpack his gun. Proud of the thing, he was. It might not match up to the finer models that some of the toffs had, but it had done him well over the years. The case was a solid one, with brass fittings. The shiny clips were lockable. He had the key on his keyring ready. But as he bent over into the boot, there was a shout from the far side of the field.

'Quick!' someone was calling. 'In the name of God! Someone get to her!'

Several members of the party began to run, and Gregory joined them, diving deep into the long grasses and sending a pheasant squealing and flapping out of the undergrowth. He saw Kenneth up ahead and then Adam Foster's tweed jacket disappearing over the embankment.

'Take care,' someone called. 'The river's high.'

When Gregory got to the edge of the field, he was just in time to see the bedraggled head of one of Adam's spaniels, bobbing in the water, and then, the current caught and swept the face out of sight. The head emerged again but much further down.

'Shit!' Adam was saying again and again. 'I'll not be able to reach her!'

Adam ran along the edge of the river, but the trees were in the way and he was forced to stop and watch in horror. Now, some of the women joined them. Rosemary was asking what had happened and when she saw, she went deathly pale and covered her mouth with her hand. Fiona was behind her.

'Who is it? Can't we do anything?' she was asking. 'Oh, don't just stand there watching, Greg. If you were a real man, you'd do something!'

Gregory elbowed his wife out of the way and bypassing Adam, ran back along the field. He knew the only chance to intercept the dog was when it came to the clearing much further along. He could hear Kenneth shouting from behind him and saw a flash of David's anxious face also.

Gregory wasn't a fit man, but spurred on now and realising that he was watched by all including Mr Dewhurst, he pumped his arms and ignored the building pain in his legs. His lungs began to ache as if they were on fire and he was forced to slow as he came to the field gate. He exited at a jog and then dived down into the brambles. His hands bled as they caught on the thorns but he crashed through shielding his face as best he could. Behind him, he heard someone follow. He came to the water's edge and looked upstream, the head that had been visible only seconds before, had disappeared completely from view. Someone was behind him now in the thicket. He didn't turn, but swore under his breath and continued to scour the water for a break in the frothing surface. He thought he spotted something and leaned out, readying himself to plunge in.

'Get a branch,' he called over his shoulder to the person behind. He heard a crashing and felt someone's hand on his back.

'Careful!' he shouted angrily, as he lost his footing and slithered. He grabbed at the bush beside him to right himself and he heard a snort. 'The branch! Pass it now! I see her coming!' he shouted, still refusing to take his eyes from the water. He reached out a hand to take it, but the branch never came. Gregory wasn't sure what happened after that. He found himself in the water and was up to his knees. His wellington boots were full and heavy with water. He cursed. Quickly, he tried to feel for the river bed beneath his feet to steady himself. The current was strong. More people were coming to the clearing where he'd fallen in. He heard Fiona's voice and another woman shouting.

Gregory began to step out to the centre of the river, feeling the water's current growing stronger and stronger as he did so. He was now almost up to his thighs. The water dragged at his clothes, urging him downstream further. He searched the bubbling surface, dragging his hands through it. He saw the animal coming closer. The river further up must have caught the body and allowed him precious time as it spun and eddied, trapped in a dense overhanging branch.

'Nearly ...' he said, and leaned further, opening his arms wide and grabbing madly at the matted hair. His hand touched it, and then hearing the roars of encouragement from the embankment, he tightened his grip, refusing to let go. But slimy and slick from the water, the hair slid from his hands, he released his loosening grip and grasped again, wildly, clenching his teeth in concentration. But he was just out of reach and the river caught and whipped the dog's head below the water and away. Gregory tried again, but it was no use. He slapped the river surface with the palm of his hand and swore loudly. He nearly lost his balance as he did so, and he was left teetering and flailing stupidly. Everything seemed to go silent. All Gregory could hear was the roar of the water in his ears.

He looked back at the crowd, gathered now on the embankment. He saw Adam shaking his head. Even Mr Dewhurst looked grief-stricken. As Gregory slowly made his way back, he saw his employer reach out and rest his hand on Adam's shoulder.

Gregory raised his arms as he neared them. 'Sorry. I did try.'

No-one spoke.

He expected to get a hand pulling himself out, but was left to scrabble his way up the steep, slippery ridge as the group dispersed. When he emerged from the brambles the mood was indeed sombre. He crossed the field without speaking. Not a word of bloody thanks from one of them. The crowd seemed to part as he approached. He looked down at his muddy wellingtons and damp trousers. A trail of pondweed, oily and green, hung from his crotch. He snatched at it and threw it to the ground in disgust. As he passed Kenneth, he was sure that the man sneered.

'Well?' Gregory said, his face growing hot. 'What's your problem then. Well? Say it now.'

Kenneth shook his head and smiled.

'Don't you dare laugh at me!' Gregory exploded. 'I've seen you, hanging around the house, trying to charm your way in with my bloody wife. Think I'm stupid, don't you?' Gregory was now inches from the other man's face. 'Well then?' he demanded.

Kenneth shook his head again and stepped aside.

'What the hell?' Fiona said, coming across now with Rosemary. 'You just can't help yourself, can you Gregory? A bloody embarrassment, that's what you are. I'd be better off with Kenny.'

He'd not have let that dog drown. You're a joke, Greg. A damn joke.'

Gregory spun round in disgust. He caught sight of the faces of all of the onlookers, many of them standing open-mouthed, holding expressions of pity and unease.

'You'll wish you'd not said that,' Gregory said quietly, refusing to look at his wife. 'You'll wish you'd not said a word.'

19

It was impossible to cancel the rest of the shoot, although it seemed that nobody was really in the mood that afternoon. But many of those participating had paid good money for the entertainment and there was a general push for the staff to jolly things along. Unsurprisingly, Adam was nowhere to be seen. Gregory overheard someone say that Mr Dewhurst had taken it upon himself to drive the distraught man up to the house for a stiff drink. Kenneth had been assigned the task of checking if, after all the crashing about and hullabaloo from earlier, there was any point in remaining where they were. After tramping the field, he announced that there was still plenty of shots to be had. Much to Gregory's disgust, he then began to organise the beaters in line and asked if anyone wanted to change pins. Bloody cheek of the man. Gregory's charges, who he now judged to be quite competent, asked if they could shoot across the river. Gregory nodded and told them that they could move.

He was left alone, for which he was glad until David ruined things and sidled up with his gun.

'Bit messy earlier,' the other man said.

Gregory grunted. David was one of the only people to have come over to speak.

'Adam was pretty cut-up. One of his finest bitches, apparently,' David went on. 'Listen, are you having a pop yourself? We were all saying over lunch that we'd not seen you shoot once. What about it? Maybe it'd cheer you a bit. I was asking Adam earlier. He said that you used a different gun to the ones the estate lends out.'

Gregory moved to the back of the Land Rover. 'You'd not catch me using one of Adam Foster's things,' he said and then froze. 'Damn it,' he cursed. 'Did I leave it like that?' The gun case was laying unlocked. He was sure he had left it sealed. He lifted the shotgun reverently, checking that it was untouched. No, it was fine after all. Must have been during all the commotion, of course. Just before Adam's dog had fallen in the river, he'd been checking the thing. Well, perhaps David was right. A shoot might indeed brighten his mood. For every bird he aimed at, he'd imagine it was bloody Fiona.

David was nodding. 'That's it, you see?' he said, smiling encouragingly. 'Maybe you can teach me a few more things. Adam was trying to get me to relax my right shoulder more. Is it right that your gun's more comfortable to hold?'

Gregory snorted and pointed. 'Doesn't help that you're shooting one of those. Over-under is best, look,' he said, holding out his own with the chamber still open for safety.

David nodded. 'It's a lot heavier. What's the real difference anyway?' He took the thing and turned it gently over.

Gregory laughed. 'Have a go with it if you like, and you'll see. Use it for the first drive. You only get two shots, but that'll focus you. I'll use your one.'

Kenneth had walked the line and checked everyone was ready. He locked eyes with Gregory. 'Well? Ready to join in this time?' he asked.

Gregory spat at the ground.

Kenneth laughed and shouted across for the beaters to begin.

There was the customary flag-waving and the exciting yelping of dogs as the line of beaters moved forwards.

David began to load the gun, his hands perhaps a little shaky, knowing that Gregory's eyes were on him.

'Oh Christ, David, no!' Gregory said, darting forward. 'Not the twenty gauge. This is a twelve. Bloody hell, that would slip down and block the barrel. If you loaded a twelve in after that, it'd explode in your face!'

The other man laughed and took the proffered ammunition.

At that moment, time seemed to stop. Gregory felt a terrible sense of foreboding. Rather than joining in with shoot as he had planned, he froze. He watched as David held the heavy gun to his shoulder and concentrated his attention. The birds came into view. A large male pheasant headed towards them.

'There you are,' Gregory shouted. 'To the left.'

David followed the flight of the flapping bird as it plunged and arced in terror.

'Now!' Gregory shouted.

The boom came.

Then silence.

He lay on the ground. It was abundantly clear to anyone who looked, that the man was quite dead.

20

'Did you hear then?' Michelle stood in the doorway, her hand on the door frame. She looked up and down the corridor in an exaggerated manner as if checking in case anyone was within earshot.

Cathy looked up from her computer. She had just been printing out a prescription at the lead receptionist's request. 'Hear what?' Cathy asked as she retrieved the prescription from the printer and checked it.

'Over the weekend. Maybe you've not been out and about much,' Michelle said, coming further into the room.

Cathy shook her head. 'I don't know what you mean.'

'Saturday evening,' Michelle went on. 'It was the talk of Glainkirk. I was out with Julie. Bit of a girls' thing. Perhaps we should have invited you.'

Cathy gave the girl a disparaging look.

Michelle laughed. 'Maybe not then. No, it was just that we were in Hudson's and the man behind the bar told us.'

Cathy put her pen down and looked sternly at Michelle.

'Right on our doorstep too. Tragedy.'

Cathy didn't ask again, but Michelle must have realised her irritation.

'A fatal shooting,' she said, shaking her head. 'Up at the farm. Sounds dreadful. An accident, so they're saying. It was at one of the big, organised shoots. Dead, and nothing they could do, apparently. Although I think the ambulance people had a shot.' The girl grimaced. 'I don't mean shot; I mean they had a go trying to revive the poor soul. Bad choice of words.'

Cathy felt suddenly cold. 'Who was killed?'

'Oh, I'm sorry. I don't know the name.'

'Man or woman?'

'It was a man, I think. Bound to have been one of those toffs that pay through the nose for a day up there. Dr Moreland, are you alright? You've gone quite pale.'

Cathy's mouth was dry. 'Yes, fine,' she stammered. 'T-thanks, Michelle, was there something else?'

'The prescription?' the girl said, stepping forward.

Cathy scrawled an unrecognisable signature and slid the paper towards her.

'Thanks,' Michelle said, moving towards the door. 'I'll let you get on. Not many house-calls as yet, so we're maybe in for a better day than Friday.'

Cathy didn't answer.

She sat for some minutes staring blankly at the computer screen. And then, rousing herself, snatched up the phone on her desk and dialled an outside line.

'Cathy?' came the reply when switchboard put her through. Suzalinna's voice was strained.

'Yes. Listen. Sorry if it's a bad time, but you were on this weekend, right?'

'You know I was. I was on day-shift because bloody Brodie's still off sick. Why?'

'A fatal shooting?'

Cathy heard her friend sigh. 'Hang on a minute, I'll shut the door.'

From the end of the line, Cathy could hear her friend moving across the room and then a thud. The phone crackled. 'OK, don't tell me this was one of yours then?' Suzalinna asked.

'I don't know,' Cathy replied. 'I only just heard. The paper-work, if there is any for me, hasn't come through yet. I've got a feeling it might well be a patient of ours though.'

After the weekend, the GPs usually received a multitude of emails and hospital correspondence letting them know of any change in their patients' conditions. The files came from the out-of-hours doctors but also regularly from the local accident and emergency department so that the GPs might know if any particular family required urgent follow-up on Monday morning.

Suzalinna was talking and from what Cathy could hear, she was also leafing through papers in her office. 'Hang on, I had it on my desk. I didn't deal with him when he came in, by the way, it was our senior registrar, Frances. I only reported it to the police when he didn't survive.'

Cathy sighed. 'It was a man then, definitely?'

'Oh yes. Had you expected someone else?'

'Sorry, no, go on,' Cathy said.

'Well, it seems that he'd been on one of these organised shoots. I assume it was all supervised correctly. God knows what went wrong. Gun backfired anyway. Ambulance was called at approximately two-thirty. To be honest, the chances of survival were pretty slim. One of the bystanders had thought he was still breathing and they started CPR. Very messy. I suppose, out of formality, the paramedics continued until he got to us. Frances called it pretty quickly, thank God, poor man. Non-shockable rhythm and he'd blown half his neck off.'

Cathy grimaced.

'So, one of yours, you think?' Suzalinna was saying. 'I've got the name somewhere.'

Cathy waited. If it was Gregory Warrender, she would never forgive herself for signing the man's form. If it was Mr Dewhurst she would always regret allowing him to shoot that day also.

Her friend spoke again. 'Here it is,' she said. 'David? A Mr David Holden. Think the police were dealing with the wife, but I suppose if he's your patient, she might warrant a visit. The estate where he was shooting will be in for a grilling, I assume.'

Cathy sighed. 'No that's fine, Suz. It's a bit of a relief really. I don't know the name. I'll check the database and see if he was ours, but he wasn't the person I was expecting you to say.'

Suzalinna laughed. 'Well, I'm glad I made your day. I was getting worried there. Thought you were mixed up in another one of your mysteries. I don't think there was anything suspicious about this man's death. Just a tragic accident. I hate gunshot wounds. Bloody messy business.' Her friend seemed to be considering and when she spoke again, her voice held a hint of warning. 'You know darling, you've had enough excitement recently to last a lifetime. Stay out of trouble, OK?'

Cathy laughed and thanking her friend, she replaced the receiver. Just an accident. Yes. It was quite alright after all. The fact that the shoot had been on the Glainkirk Farm Estate had admittedly made her twitchy, but she had no reason to worry at all. An unfortunate accident. That was all.

Gregory Warrender sighed dramatically. It had been a dreadful twenty-four hours and his mood, already black, was only worsened when Fiona announced that she was going to ask Rosemary to come and stay.

'It's a stupid idea. Why not go to hers and stay over?' he asked. Their house was far too small to accommodate a grieving widow and he knew that he for one, was completely socially incompetent in dealing with such an unusual situation.

'Don't be so heartless,' Fiona had retorted. 'It's the offer more than anything. No doubt her family will want to have her. They live somewhere down south, I think. Of course, she can't stay in that house alone. Not the house they lived in together. All those memories and photographs everywhere. It would be awful.'

Gregory shrugged. 'What about work?' He didn't care much about Fiona's employers but he supposed they must at least warrant an explanation for both Rosemary and Fiona's absence if that was what his wife was suggesting.

'I called earlier. Didn't you hear? I told them I was taking the week off in case she needed me. They were very understanding, as it happens. They'd already heard all about it so I assume Rosemary had spoken to them before.'

Gregory snorted. No doubt if they were so accommodating, it posed the question as to whether his wife's job was really that necessary. A whole week off and no concern only meant that you were surplus to requirements anyway.

'I need to get on,' he said, moving to the door.

'I might not be at home for some of the day if I'm going to Glainkirk to sit with Rosemary.'

'Well, I can't drive you,' Gregory said.

'I'll get a lift from someone.'

Gregory shot his wife a look, knowing only too well what this might mean. But he was in no mood to have his suspicions confirmed. Bloody Kenneth would be in his element no doubt. Well, the pair were welcome to one another.

'When will you be back?' Fiona asked.

He didn't answer. How was he meant to know anyway? The farm wasn't a nine-to-five, that was if he still had a job at the end of the day. Gregory made his way to the jeep. Although he hadn't admitted it to Fiona, he had slept dreadfully the night before. In the early hours of the morning, he had given up tossing and turning and had gone to the back door to stand and breath in the night air. The sky had been clear and the moon an ice-white. He had stood there in the freezing cold, his breath a bitter haze, clouding in front of his face. As he stood, he went over the day's events and wondered for the hundredth time, what on earth had happened.

Gregory was no fool. The thought that the gun had been tampered with had not escaped his mind. And if this was so, where did that leave him? He recalled his surprise on returning to the boot of the Land Rover only to find the gun case unlocked. Had he really left it like that before the commotion over Adam Foster's stupid dog? Gregory tried to remember. He visualised the shiny brass catches on the gun case and his hands on them with the set of keys. But it was no use. For the life of him, he couldn't be sure. And what did it matter anyway? If he hadn't left the thing open, then he had been thoughtless enough to leave the keys lying in the boot. How easy it must have been to simply unlock the thing while the group's attention was on the river. How simple to remove the gun. But why might anyone want to do such a thing?

Gregory thought hard. His face screwed up in concentration. If the gun had been tampered with as he suspected, then it could only mean one thing. Someone had meant the firearm to explode in his face. Only a chance comment from David had meant that the guns were switched at the final moment. Gregory had intended to shoot that afternoon. Everyone knew that. If he had used the gun instead of David, the inevitable result would have been his own death.

But unable to adjust to this realisation, and suddenly realising he was frozen through, Gregory had closed the back door and moved around the kitchen. He didn't want to wake Fiona so he shut the kitchen door and only then flicked on the lights so that he might make himself a mug of hot coffee. More to warm his hands on than anything else. As he waited for the kettle to boil, he was unable to prevent himself from seeing again the prostrate figure lying at his feet. David's head and neck had been thrown back by the force of the explosion. His throat was bloodied. Gregory refused to focus on the face, which was quite unrecognisable. The neck, he managed. He stared, unable to look away. For some reason, he was fixated by the crisp line of David's white shirt collar and the approaching seepage of deep red. Gregory wasn't sure how long he had stood motionless, but he felt strong hands on his shoulders and staggered backwards and away, nearly falling as he did so. Time seemed to be frozen. Men were shouting and he watched in a daze as they tried to help. Someone yelled that they thought David was still breathing.

Gregory had seen death before though. He had surveyed the angle of the broken neck of a pheasant enough times to recognise that David was beyond help. Still, they persisted. Someone must have phoned for an ambulance. Adam Foster was there, although Gregory had no idea from where he had appeared or when. He saw too, Mr Dewhurst, standing well back from the scene. The old gentleman seemed to have aged further than when Gregory had last seen him. He had glanced across in Gregory's direction and hastily turned away. Did he blame Gregory in some way?

It was only after the ambulance left, carrying the injured man away, blue lights illuminating the stark country lanes, that certainty hit Gregory.

'Well?' Adam asked him. 'What the hell happened?'

Gregory gaped in disbelief at the man's attitude, his power over Adam, long forgotten.

Mr Dewhurst came over too and said something quietly to his estate manager. Adam moved away and, in the distance, Gregory was aware of him herding up the shooters and beaters, and ushering them into their Land Rovers.

The old man still stood by Gregory's side. 'The police will be involved,' he said. His voice cracked.

Gregory looked at Mr Dewhurst in astonishment. 'The p-police?' he stammered.

The old man nodded and looked away, watching as the first of the cars moved slowly out of the field.

'The gun he was using. It wasn't one of ours. Adam said it was your own.'

Gregory went to speak, but his mouth seemed to be full of cotton-wool.

'Anyway,' Mr Dewhurst said, still scanning the peripheries of the field. 'I expect to see you in the estate office on Monday morning first thing. No doubt we'll have news from the hospital by then. He was an acquaintance of yours? Family in the area?'

Gregory swallowed. 'Family?' he asked, and then realising what the old man meant; 'A wife. She was here at lunchtime. My own wife's friend.'

Mr Dewhurst nodded. 'Yes. Of course, she'll need to be informed.'

'Yes,' Gregory repeated. 'Yes. I suppose she will.'

The old man stooped and picked up the gun that had caused the damage. 'Perhaps I should ...'

'Yes,' Gregory said, unsure of what the procedure was in these circumstances.

To look at the firearm, no-one might imagine the damage it had caused only minutes before. As the old man turned it over though, Gregory saw the side of one barrel completely blown out. A seared rupture of metal, twisted and cracked from the force.

'Blocked barrel,' Mr Dewhurst stated.

'Yes.'

'You checked it beforehand?'

'I did.'

The old man held the gun as if it was the filthiest thing he had ever touched.

'Well. As I say, we'll see if the man survives and then we'll know what we're dealing with.'

Gregory tried to swallow but something seemed lodged in his throat. He coughed and was afraid he was going to disgrace himself and cry in front of Mr Dewhurst. But the old man was moving away. The field was now quite deserted, other than the last Land Rover full of shooters which was now slowly making its way to the gate.

Gregory looked away, unable to watch the old man leave.

When he was sure that Mr Dewhurst was far enough away, he dropped to his haunches and took great gulps of air, as if breathing it in for the first time. His lungs hurt with every inhalation and his temples pounded. He wondered if he was going to faint. Please God, not before Mr Dewhurst was out of sight completely. Gregory touched the damp grass, trying to find stability in the earth. Hot tears brimmed at his eyes and he shook his head angrily. But beneath his fingers, he felt something uneven and hard. He shifted his hand and looked down. There, in amongst the grasses, partly covered by loose dirt, was something shining. Gregory gave this his full attention. Mesmerised, he picked the thing up and looked at it in amazement. Gregory turned it over in the palm of his hand, his self-pity now abated. The object was twisted and the metal surface battered, but it was unmistakable.

Gregory instinctively snatched it into his hand and drove his fist deep into his jacket pocket.

Mr Dewhurst was by his jeep at the far side of the field. 'Monday morning,' the old man shouted across to him.

Well, it's Monday morning now, Gregory thought, looking up at the clock. Since he had spoken to Mr Dewhurst last, David's death had been confirmed. Only time would tell how things might progress.

22

R osemary looked at her hands. What was she meant to do now? Fiona was talking but she hadn't heard a thing. She smiled at her fingertips and nodded. Perhaps she should have done as the police officer had suggested and made an appointment with her GP. Something to help her sleep, the young uniformed man had said. She had barely managed an hour's rest alone in their double bed the previous night. She couldn't go on like this forever. They had also suggested she go to stay with someone so as not to be alone in the house but, how could she? Her parents were in London and who else was there? Certainly not Fiona and Gregory, although the girl had suggested it.

Fiona was keeping up her monologue of sympathy. It fell on deaf ears. Rosemary instinctively glanced at the mantlepiece and the collection of photographs. A suited David smiled back at her, a smart but casual David, lowered his sunglasses and winked at her. Rosemary shivered and rubbed her forearm, feeling the prickle of hairs. She found herself transfixed for a moment by a photograph of him on his first day at work. His job at the estate agents had seen him rise quickly in the firm's estimation. So proud he had been, and so full of hope.

Rosemary was aware that she had been asked a question. She looked across at her young friend. If it hadn't been for that silly shoot, David might still be alive, sitting here with her, talking down to her in his slightly teasing way. She shifted in her chair.

'I'm quite alright,' she reassured Fiona, for the umpteenth time. But this again set her off on another rambling commiseration, and Rosemary was able to retreat into her thoughts once more.

She knew that she would not be financially hard up. Bless David, for all his boastfulness, he had at least done right by her in that way. She might well take a short break from work and adjust to widowhood. Her employers, especially Alfie Greyson, had been hugely sympathetic on the phone. They had told her to take as long as was needed. Rosemary looked at the vase by the window; overflowing with beautiful white flowers, a gift from the office staff. In some ways, it might be a relief to be back there in the thick of things.

Rosemary smiled sadly and wondered if she was really to blame? She had, after all, encouraged the meal, and then, when the shoot was mentioned, it had been her that had smoothed that over too. It had been what David had wanted, but it still seemed her fault.

Rosemary cast her mind back to the fated evening only days before. Gregory had been outright rude to both her and David. Rosemary had met the man on several occasions in the past when he had picked Fiona up from the railway station. She hadn't found him as bad at these times, but certainly, the other evening he seemed resolute to upset and embarrass Fiona in front of her guests.

David had agreed with this sentiment when she brought it up later.

'Don't much care how rude the fool is,' David had laughed as he undressed that evening having arrived home following the dreadful meal. He stepped out of his suit trousers and lay them over the back of a chair beside the bed.

Rosemary went to the bathroom, but David's voice had followed her.

'Stroke of genius, you organising the thing, Rose. God knows how I never thought of the thing myself. Doubt the brochures will go anywhere other than their kitchen bin though, but it was always unlikely.'

He had appeared in the doorway wearing only his pink shirt and boxer shorts. Rosemary, who had been removing her makeup, looked disparagingly at him in the mirror.

'Everything seems to have an agenda with you,' she had accused.

'Well darling,' he said, coming across the room and grasping her waist from behind. 'You don't think I went to have dinner with them just for the fun of it, did you?'

Rosemary turned on him savagely. 'Fiona is my friend,' she said, removing his hands from her hips. 'You came because of me. You were showing your support for me.' She had spun back to the mirror, her face pale.

David had playfully slapped her on the bottom and returned to the bedroom. Rosemary stood furiously clutching the basin until her anger had subsided. It was true, David did always have an underlying agenda. Perhaps in marrying her, she had been part of his big scheme. Rosemary had given up so much. She had left behind her family, not that it had been much of a tear, to be honest, given that her mother was a frightful moan. But she had moved to follow David's dream. Time and again, they had chased a new vision he had. When Rosemary married, she had come from a wealthy enough upbringing. She thought perhaps that her father's business acumen had been what had attracted David to her in the first place. Rosemary had sat silently listening to the pair of them laughing together during their first few months of marriage. Her father enjoyed David's puppyish adoration and only encouraged him more. Rosemary sometimes glanced across the table at her mother, but she had a quite different expression. Sometimes Rosemary wondered if her mother outright hated David, but they never spoke of it and she never understood why. Perhaps back then, the older woman realised that David had loved the lifestyle rather than the person he married. How funny though that he should be the one with all the airs and graces, when in fact he had originated from infinitely more humble beginnings than she.

When she had come back through from the bathroom that evening following the meal, he was in bed.

'Come on Rose, you knew why we were going. I told you. Don't be such a sourpuss, there's a good girl,' he had said, looking up from the television. He had the football scores on and he hardly noticed her reaction as she slid into bed beside him. As she lay her head on the pillow, listening to his jubilant reaction on seeing that his team had won, she had questioned David's genuine commitment to her. At the time, she had put this down to overtiredness. But now, nothing seemed clear.

Rosemary cast her mind back to the last time she had seen to her husband. The lunchtime of the shoot. He had been in high spirits having apparently spoken to Adam Foster all that morning. Triumphant didn't even come close to describing it. Over lunch, she had watched him all smiles, chatting away with the estate team as if they were great friends. If his company did succeed in what he proposed, all of the farmworkers might lose their jobs. It was sickeningly hypocritical of David to chum up to any of them, when he was their enemy, although, of course, none of them could know that. Yes. It was all rather disgusting in a way to think of it now and David had, of course, only been hours away from death. Oh God, it was too frightful to even think about.

At least he had gone, doing something he loved. That was what someone had said to her. She couldn't remember who. So many people had spoken to her. It was little consolation though. The remark, in fact, seemed quite insensitive. Probably Fiona had said it. The girl was looking at her quizzically now.

'What was that?' she asked, her voice slightly phlegmy.

'It was just, I was saying that it doesn't make any sense,' Fiona said. 'Gregory is usually so careful over his gun. I hope you don't blame him for David's death. Oh, Rosemary! Please say that you don't. I can't imagine what could have possibly happened. I know we were all joking around at lunchtime, do you remember? Someone said something a little mean about David's technique and then someone else mentioned the other type of gun as being better for him. Do you think that's what happened? David wanted to try a different gun? I don't remember now who said it, but I wish they hadn't. Otherwise, why did David have the gun in the first place? None of it makes any sense at all.'

Rosemary's mouth set in a firm line. 'No,' she said quietly. 'None of it makes any sense.'

23

Gregory looked from Adam to Mr Dewhurst and back again. What did they expect him to say? He didn't know the first thing about David, or his business. Why were they so determined to suggest that he did? Gregory swallowed twice and then fiddled with the top button on his shirt.

'I didn't know him, exactly,' he finally said and then lapsed into obstinate silence once more.

The old gentleman crossed to the window of the office and looked out. Gregory wondered what he was staring at so intently. He found himself following Mr Dewhurst's gaze and even from his seated position, Gregory could make out the tops of the trees, swaying in the wind. He wished that he was outside, gulping in the cool, gusty breeze, riding his tractor with the window open and the fields limitless before him.

Gregory licked his lips. He thought about saying something again. He was just preparing himself when Mr Dewhurst spun around and faced him once more. The old man's weathered cheeks were florid and his eyes narrow. Gregory turned away. He found himself looking at Adam, who sat across the desk, impassive and superior. Gregory hated bloody Adam Foster more than ever. He scowled and scuffed the side of his shoe against the leg of the chair.

Gregory was in no doubt that the debacle that weekend had come as a victory for the estate manager. Another opportunity to belittle Gregory and make himself look more significant. Of course, no-one could pretend that the accident wouldn't impact on the shooting business. That was bad for all the employees, especially given what Gregory had heard about Mr Dewhurst's financial state of play. Still, Gregory thought, without a doubt, Adam had a look of triumph about him. The cheek of it, especially after what Gregory had done, in risking his own life, diving into the river to retrieve the man's nasty spaniel. He wished he could tell Mr Dewhurst about his estate manager's indiscretion over the accounts. How might the old man react knowing that someone he trusted more than any was doing the dirty behind his back? Gregory wondered if he should come out with it now before they accused him of anything else. Without question, it would lead to Adam's dismissal. But then, Gregory wasn't so sure he wanted that just yet. In realizing Adam's secret, Gregory held a position of power that he was still to enjoy. He knew also, that although Adam was playing the game, going along with what Mr Dewhurst was saying, he must surely see that if Gregory was fired, he too might face the chop. Gregory would hardly go without taking Adam with him. The smarmy man must know that. No, Gregory felt sure that if push came to shove, Adam would do everything he possibly could to ensure his safety.

Although all of this was true, Gregory was still afraid. He was no fool, but they were cleverer than him. If there was a way of attributing blame without injuring themselves, they would find it. Let stupid, dumb Gregory take the rap to save their own necks. He would have to tread very carefully indeed if he was to escape difficulty, that was for sure.

But Mr Dewhurst was now pacing the room, his hands clasped behind his back. Gregory was reminded of his old headmaster. On one occasion as a boy, he had visited the man's office for spitting in the corridor. He was given the belt for that. Gregory shifted in his seat, remembering the sting of the strap on his legs. At least Mr Dewhurst couldn't physically assault him, although, by the look of him, he might dearly like to.

'Well? He was your guest,' Mr Dewhurst said. 'You must know something about this David Holden. Adam says he was a last-minute addition. What was it all about then?'

'I'd hardly spoken to him before. It was my wife really. She and his wife were friends. They work together in the office. They came to our house for a meal the night before. He was trying to peddle one of his new-builds to us, I think. I wouldn't entertain the idea, but Fiona was all over it. He brought a brochure to the house when he came, and said he was interested in the shooting, that was all. He'd shot before, but only clays.'

Mr Dewhurst shook his head in disgust and turned to Adam.

'I'm afraid, Gregory, that it seems your friend had more than a superficial interest in the estate's business,' he said quietly.

Gregory gaped stupidly.

'A number of chance remarks during the shoot led me to do a bit of digging last night,' Adam said. The estate manager sighed. 'He worked for Oliver and Treadwell, the agents in town.'

Gregory still didn't understand.

'It seems that your friend had designs on Glainkirk Farm Estate,' Adam said.

'What?' asked Gregory, completely confused. 'I knew he was an estate agent, but how could he afford to buy the farm?'

Adam rolled his eyes and glanced at Mr Dewhurst. The old

man looked as if Gregory was something foul and smelly on the sole of his shoe.

'He didn't want to buy it for himself, you fool. He was wanting the land. To take over and manage the place as part of the agents' portfolio initially, but I suspect the real idea was to build on it. Some grand scheme about new houses for commuters. Had us in his sights for a while. He wrote to me a few months ago. Tossed the letter in the bin without a second thought. I wouldn't have agreed to what he was suggesting ever,' the old man said.

Adam nodded.

Gregory looked from one man to the other. So that's what the devious man had been after. He had made a comment over the meal that night. Gregory might have guessed. If David had pulled his nasty scheme off, it would have spelt the end to his farm. Gregory thought of his cattle and clenched his fists.

'We've still to get to the bottom of how he had your gun too,' Mr Dewhurst said. 'You surely know the rules by now. God knows you've worked for us long enough. Adam always sorts guns for the less experienced guests. It's done for everyone's safety. The estate guns are checked thoroughly. Adam does it himself along with the paperwork. He assigns each guest their own numbered gun. They're insured.' The old man turned away and raised a hand to his forehead. 'Christ alone knows if we're covered for this man blowing his brains out using another gun.'

Adam grimaced.

'My gun was checked too. Adam, you were a character reference. My GP. I saw Dr Moreland. She signed the ...' But he could see that there was little he could say to appease them.

Mr Dewhurst turned to Adam. 'What have the people said about it so far? I assume you've called?'

'I left a message with the insurers this morning, of course,' Adam said. 'I'm waiting to hear back. I don't know how they'll handle it. Probably need to wait for a more official inquiry. I think we'll need to approach the man's widow and see if we can placate any potentially harmful feelings. Be as supportive and approachable as possible, I'd say.'

Mr Dewhurst nodded. 'Yes. Yes, of course. Send some flowers or something.'

Adam jotted this down in his notebook. 'The police will no doubt want to come back,' he said.

'Police?' Gregory interrupted. 'Have they been then?'

'Yes, Mr Warrender,' Mr Dewhurst said, his voice heavy with sarcasm. 'Do you honestly think a fatal shooting would escape their interest?' The old man snorted. 'I've had them up at the house most of yesterday evening. Took your gun away with them,' he said. 'Thankfully the local constabulary isn't exactly known for their tenacity. I think I dealt with it as best I could, but they'll be back. Without a doubt, they'll need to speak to you, given that it was your gun, and that you were in charge of supervising its bloody use.'

Mr Dewhurst face had turned a mottled shade of purple.

Gregory's tongue stuck to the roof of his mouth. 'I checked it,' he said. 'He was going to put the wrong cartridge in. I stopped him just in time. The barrel was empty.'

'You can say all that to the police,' the old man retorted. 'Dirt, I presume. Must have got stuck deep in the barrel and the build-up caused the thing to backfire. Bloody mess. No-one should have to witness that. On my estate too. Renowned for our good safety record. Damn joke it is. A damned disgrace.'

'It wasn't full of dirt,' Gregory persisted. 'I kept my gun clean.'

But it was clear that Mr Dewhurst wasn't listening. The old man moved towards the door of the office.

'I'll be up at the house, Adam. I'll have my mobile if you

need to contact me. If the police do arrive unannounced, let me know, and if you hear about the insurers ...'

Adam nodded. 'Yes, of course. I'll see that you know at once. Thank you.'

Mr Dewhurst placed his hand on the door handle. 'For now,' he said to Gregory. 'You remain an employee. That's thanks to Adam here. I'd have given you your marching orders this morning if it hadn't been for his guidance. Count yourself lucky. But you're on borrowed time, Mr Warrender. If it does turn out that you are, even in the smallest portion, liable for the man's death...' He didn't finish his sentence but instead left the room, slamming the door as he went.

Gregory and Adam sat in silence, listening to the retreating footsteps on the gravel outside.

When it was clear that Mr Dewhurst was well out of earshot, Adam leaned back in his chair and smiled.

'Well then, Greg. Care to tell me exactly how you went about murdering him then?'

24

'Dr Moreland, hello. I must apologise for disturbing you when you must be busy at work.' The line crackled and Cathy waited with the receiver to her ear. 'This isn't a professional call about my health, Doctor. The tablets that you prescribed me are fine. No, it's something rather more delicate I'm afraid. I assume you have time to talk just now?'

Cathy glanced up at the clock on the wall.

'Yes, I have time, what is it I can do?'

There was a pause. 'Tricky really and I'm sorry to ask. You'll no doubt have heard the news? It seems to have spread all over town, and no wonder in many ways. The shooting on the estate this weekend? I seem to remember you suggesting that I didn't go for the sake of my health. I'll conjecture that another man might well have benefited from that advice, but God alone knows what happened. It's too late now anyway.'

'I heard, yes. A fatal shooting. It was an accident though surely?'

She heard the old man snort. 'My first thought also. The gun backfired. I assumed that it had been a case of poor gun maintenance, but I'm now beginning to wonder ...'

'I don't understand,' Cathy said, with a dreadful sinking feeling.

'No, I'm afraid that I'm not explaining myself terribly well. It's been a shock. I had the police at the house all yesterday evening. They will do their own little investigation of course. It would have been a simple matter, had the gun in question been one belonging to the estate. Well, when I say simple, I mean, we'd have been covered insurance-wise, if you see what I mean? Sadly, it's not that straightforward. It is a sport with its dangers I suppose. Accidents do happen, admittedly infrequently, but it might well be put down as such.'

'I sense a 'but' coming,' Cathy said.

'Well, then you are correct, Dr Moreland. There is a 'but' and a big one. The gun wasn't one of ours. The unfortunate man had been lent an estate shotgun at the beginning of the shoot. We check them over carefully and they are all in excellent order. But it appears that the man swapped it for another, on the afternoon shoot. I've still no idea why it happened, but there it is. One of our farmhands was on the shoot that day and he brought his own gun. That's quite alright, as long as they have paperwork to prove it's been licensed correctly – which he had. He, and the man who died, apparently knew one another. It seems that the farmhand arranged for the man to join the shoot only that morning, very much at the last minute.'

She waited.

'You're probably still wondering why I called. Yes, I can see that.'

Cathy heard him sigh.

'It's just that I have a horrible suspicion that there's more to this accident than meets the eye.'

'The police ...'

'Oh yes, the local constabulary will analyse the gun, no doubt. They are doing exactly that now, I believe. What they will find is anyone's guess, but I'd be willing to put money on them discovering that it had been tampered with.'

Cathy was speechless. She tried to form a response but instead found her saliva catching at the back of her throat. She coughed.

'Dr Moreland?' came the old man's voice.

'Yes, I'm still here. A bit taken aback I must admit. Why, if you don't mind me asking, would you think that this wasn't an accidental death?'

'My estate manager has done a bit of digging. He's competent and resourceful. The man who died had designs on my land. He worked for the local land and estate agents. They had been tentatively putting out feelers to see if I might sell up. But more than that, the man who's gun he borrowed has begun to give me cause for concern. He is a loyal employee, to be honest with you. Very hard working and, from what the estate manager tells me, the job is more to him than that. It's a vocation. Warrender's my lead cattleman and damn good at what he does. Comes from a farming background, although with no land in the family he was destined to find labouring jobs. Been with the estate for several years and no bother from him.'

So, Gregory Warrender was involved after all. Cathy's stomach flipped. She tried to be rational though. What Mr Dewhurst implied didn't make any sense.

'I assume you're suggesting that he deliberately did something to his gun and then handed it over knowing it might kill? But why? Why would he risk his job and his life?'

'Well, that's just it. If he knew about the risk to the land, it makes you wonder. I've had an interview with him down at the office. Shifty to say the least and not an answer for anything. You see, if my estate manager is correct and this man loves his job so much, could he bear the thought of the land being sold?'

'I see. It does seem a little extreme, doesn't it?'

'Well, that's as may be. These rustic sorts can be ardent over their cause though. I must tell you that he had no reason for concern. I have absolutely no intention of selling my estate over to developers. The thought makes my blood boil. Horrible, boxy, new houses being put up all over my family's land? It would be like selling my soul to the devil himself.'

'I still don't see how I can be of help.'

'I did just wonder, you see?' Mr Dewhurst said. 'It was after your senior partner had mentioned your interest in things of this sort. The police are all well and good, but an educated, sensitive approach may be more suitable.'

Cathy looked skyward. 'Mr Dewhurst ...' she began, but he interrupted.

'The other point I should have stated is that the man who I suspect of arranging this whole gun debacle is apparently well-known to you.'

Cathy dreaded what was coming.

'A Mr Gregory Warrender. You signed off his gun licence only last week it seems. Well, Doctor? If it turns out that he was responsible, it does put you also in a difficult spot. Should you have signed the form in the first place?'

Cathy swallowed but didn't speak.

'Oh, I don't want to sound overbearing,' the old man continued, 'but I assume you'd rather be in on this, than outside, looking in? What do you say then, Dr Moreland? It's imperative to my reputation that this fiasco is cleared up swiftly and sensitively. Will you help?'

25

Cathy sat for some moments after replacing the telephone receiver. Her gut feeling about Gregory Warrender had been right all along. He had been involved.

Having no mobile number in the notes, Cathy tried to call the last recorded house number, secretly hoping that she would get Fiona rather than her husband, although, what she was going to say, she wasn't quite sure. The phone rang out. Of course, it was a Monday. Fiona had mentioned that she worked in Forkieth in an office during the week. Cathy checked the computer and saw that there was a house visit waiting to be seen. If she took it, she might still have time to drive up to the Warrenders before returning to the practice.

The roads in Glainkirk were surprisingly quiet. When, typically, shoppers might spill out onto the high street, the place seemed quite deserted. She drove, lost in her thoughts. The sound from the radio irritated her and she flicked it off, preferring silence.

The day was overcast. Puddles that had been iced over first-thing, had thawed and as she accelerated, she heard the repetitive swish of tyre in water. She reached the house she was after far faster than she might have otherwise and parked poorly, too distracted to notice. An informal courtyard extended allowing access to the small bungalows, each of which displayed a handrail and ramp to the door. As she got out, the cold air stung her face. She grabbed her bag and notes and jogged across the tarmac. Waiting, she stamped her feet on the doorstep to keep warm.

Mr Duncan must have seen her from the window but it still took him an age to get to the door.

'Come through,' he said, turning and leading the way slowly into the carpeted hallway. 'That's it, shut it after you. I can feel that wind right through to my bones today. I was glad when I saw your car. Didn't fancy one of the new ones coming out.'

Cathy smiled to herself, and obeyed the instruction, pulling both the front door and the inner glass one shut behind. 'How have you been?' she asked, trying to put her other concerns from her head. 'I was worried when I saw you'd put in a call for today.'

She saw the man's hunched shoulders sag a little.

'Not so good recently?' she asked. 'Perhaps I should have been out sooner?'

Mr Duncan turned and Cathy saw for the first time that his eyes were moist.

'Oh, dear. Shall we have a sit-down and you can tell me what's been going on?'

Mr Duncan was well-known to the practice. His wife had died some years before and he had struggled, growing gradually more infirm himself. None of his own medical complaints were life-threatening. Mild to moderate osteoarthritis, reasonably-controlled hypertension, recurrent gout. Cathy knew that he was the kind of patient who might well have benefited from the traditional kind of general practice, with his family doctor visiting weekly, just to see how he was. These days, however, the GPs had little time for such indulgences. But Mr Duncan was undoubtedly faltering. The last time Cathy had been out, she had asked the community care manager to pop in past and see if he might warrant some extra services. When there was little medically wrong, her hands were tied.

Cathy sat on the stiff-backed sofa and smiled sympathetically. If she finished up here fast, she might still have time to pop up to Glainkirk Farm and see if Fiona Warrender was at home. She really must find out what had happened with Gregory's gun, and make sure the girl was safe also. She thought of the bruise on Fiona's arm. Now, her husband was suspected of involvement in another man's death, what else was he capable of? And how on earth had Cathy allowed herself to miss the red flags? Why had she allowed Fiona to leave her consultation room without addressing the concern she had over the bruise? And why had she signed Gregory's form? If Mr Dewhurst raised the question, then the police must surely do so also. Cathy glanced at the clock on the mantlepiece. She should make it if she was quick before afternoon surgery started.

Mr Duncan was fussing, sitting himself down and adjusting the cushions on the chair behind. He tutted several times in annoyance at his inability to get the arrangement right. Cathy saw that his face was mottled and she glanced down at his ankles, wondering if his heart might be failing. Often swelling of the lower extremities was the first sign.

'I can't really complain,' he was saying, shaking his head. 'It's just I've been having a bad week.'

'How so?' Cathy asked, but she knew the answer.

He nodded slightly and then rooted in his trouser pocket for a large cotton handkerchief. The cloth was heavily creased and he pressed it to his face and sighed, his breath coming in a shuddering gasp.

'I'm sorry it's still so difficult,' she told him, filling the silence so that he was able to compose himself. 'We spoke about a tablet to help, if you remember? I know you were reluctant before, but I think it's worth consideration. I was telling you about the newer medications. They have few side-effects and don't make you woozy.'

He was shaking his head.

'Your mood?' she asked quickly. 'Is it like this all the time?'

Mr Duncan shrugged. 'I don't know what to say.'

'If you're miserable all the time, wouldn't you try taking something to help?'

He shook his head again.

Cathy felt exasperated. If he took a small dose of an antidepressant, he might well notice a difference. His days alone and miserable must seem to extend on into eternity, and without his beloved wife, it was like never-ending torture. She tried again. 'Honestly,' she said. 'I wish you'd trust me. I do know my job. Believe me, I've seen enough people going through this. How many times have I been out to see you over the years now? You're no better than when Mary just died.'

Her words landed into stunned silence and she wished she could take them back almost at once. Too harsh, she thought, watching the man's face crumple in embarrassment.

'I'm sorry if it came out wrong,' she said hurriedly. 'I didn't mean to sound offensive. Of course, I don't mind at all coming to see you, Mr Duncan. It's frustrating that I can see a way to help and you won't take it.'

Again, she felt she'd got it wrong. The elderly man nodded but didn't look at her.

'Look, I can't force the tablets on you,' she said, glancing at the clock. 'Would you at least think about what I've said? It's hard to see you like this every time I visit. It's heartbreaking to watch.'

Mr Duncan seemed to finally rouse himself. He exhaled and placed his hands on his knees. 'I'll let you know if I change my mind. Thank you so much for coming out to visit today. I'm sorry if I've been a nuisance.'

Cathy laughed, but he didn't smile. 'Please Mr Duncan, you know I didn't mean that at all. I'm terribly sorry if I've spoken out of turn. Please forgive me. I've had a lot on my mind recently. I'll go, but I'd like to ring you later in the week perhaps, to see how you are. Could I do that?'

The old man was getting up. He moved to the living-room door and held onto it, steadying himself.

'I'll let you get on.'

Guilt anchored in her stomach as she rose and crossed the room. Mr Duncan, who would usually have waved her off at the door until she was out of sight, remained rooted to the spot.

When Cathy got into her car, she swore loudly. Oh God, what a mess. She'd phone him later and apologise once again. Honestly, it was so hard.

As she drove out the sheltered housing court, she glanced in the rearview mirror and saw the curtain in Mr Duncan's front window move. Well, what was she meant to do, if the man wouldn't help himself? An antidepressant had been a reasonable suggestion. If he took offence at it, then really, there was nothing more she could do about the thing. She had only been trying to help after all.

Cathy checked the time. Yes, she'd still get there and back if she was quick. She'd forego lunch and should make it back to the practice if she hurried. Cathy signalled and turned left onto the road that led out of town and towards Glainkirk Farm Estate.

26

By the time Cathy arrived, it was gone one o'clock. She parked her car in a grassy area that looked like it had been used for that very purpose previously and got out. Although she had never visited before, she felt sure that she must be in the right place.

The house was in darkness, which of course wasn't surprising given the time of day, but it did make her heart sink. It was set back off the track and sheltered by a small copse of sycamore trees which, had it been summer, might have cast a gentle dappled effect across the lawn in front. Instead, the bare branches were stark reminders of the season and projected like desperate hands to the sky. Cathy glanced up and feeling a sudden chill, wrapped her jacket more tightly around herself and crossed the track. She pushed the metal gate noting that it needed oiling and walked up the path to the front door. For some reason, she suddenly felt quite nervous. Ridiculous really. She had done thousands of house visits over the years and she had every reason to be there. Both Gregory and Fiona Warrender were, after all, her patients and following Mr

Dewhurst's telephone call, it was entirely appropriate for her to be concerned for their welfare.

Cathy hesitated on the doorstep before summoning up the courage to knock. Holding her breath, she listened for any movement inside. It soon became clear that if anyone was home, they weren't coming to the door.

Cathy shivered again and realising that she was now quite cold through, she retraced her steps. As she did so, she became aware of a car engine. The sound seemed to echo up the lane and then despite the time of day, the headlights came into view. Cathy hovered uncertainly, not wanting to be caught snooping, but eager to speak with anyone to ask after the Warrenders. The car approached, coming rapidly up the bumpy track towards her. She wondered at first if it was going to stop, but it slowed and then came the inevitable rasp of loose gravel as the wheels spun. The pickup parked behind her own car. Cathy still stood by the Warrenders' garden gate.

A man got out. Cathy didn't recognise him. He crossed the lane in a purposeful, relaxed manner. His hair was dark and slightly curly and it seemed likely that he was an employee of the estate given his attire. He smiled and Cathy instinctively liked him. She felt her shoulders relax.

'Alright?' he asked. 'Lost?'

Cathy found herself blushing. 'No,' she said. 'I was looking for the Warrenders. I think I'm in the right place? It's so hard to tell in the country. No numbers on people's doors.'

The man laughed. 'Yes, that's true. You're in the right place though, but Greg will be up at the cattle, and Fi's out for the day.'

Cathy nodded, noting the man's informal reference to Mrs Warrender.

'Of course,' she said. She glanced behind him. 'I'll perhaps try them again another time. I thought I might be taking a chance coming out anyway. I wanted to check in and see how they were.'

'Friend of the family?' the man asked, resting his hand on the gate.

Cathy looked down and saw that there were several deep scratches on his knuckles. The man looked down too.

'Hazard of the job,' he laughed. 'So, you know them well?'

Cathy hesitated, wondering how to reply. 'In a way, yes,' she said.

He smiled disarmingly again. 'Well, if it helps, I know where Fi is. I dropped her off earlier in town. She's visiting a friend. Poor woman's only just lost her husband this weekend.'

'Oh dear,' Cathy said. 'How dreadful.'

'Yes,' he agreed. 'Terrible accident, and on our shoot too. Doesn't look good for the estate, and we're usually so careful. But the man shouldn't have been there at all it seems. Wasn't on the list anyway.' He glanced at Cathy. 'He was invited at the last minute by Greg, as it happens,' he explained. 'Not sure what went wrong. The gun went off in the poor chap's face. Didn't stand much of a chance.'

'How horrible.'

'It's shaken us all up a bit, I can tell you. But of course, Fi's friend, the man's wife, will be in a terrible state today. That's why she went over.'

'I see,' Cathy said. 'Yes. I see.'

Cathy smiled at the man. Mr Dewhurst's words were still heavy in her thoughts. *You signed the gun licence. Well, Doctor?* Perhaps she was being horribly selfish, but would she be held accountable if it transpired that Gregory had indeed caused the man's death? If it came to it, she still couldn't answer why exactly she had been so easily swayed. Had it been because he had done her a favour in dragging her car from a ditch? Cathy had thought of her general practice revalidation papers still sitting waiting to be completed in her spare bedroom at home and swallowed.

The man was looking at her in a puzzled sort of way. Realising that she must have been staring blankly at him, she began to move to her car. 'Thanks,' she said as she passed. 'I'll pop back another time.'

As Cathy settled herself in her car, ready to return to the practice, she wondered who he was and what impact his presence might have had on Fiona's marriage.

Cathy reversed and turned the car in the small lane. As she drove towards the main road, she thought of the good-looking man. Yes. He might well cause cracks in what already seemed to be a fragile marriage, that was certain. Despite the reassurance that Fiona was safe visiting a friend, Cathy experienced a dreadful sense of foreboding as she returned to Glainkirk.

27

G regory had had a hard-enough day as it was. The final nail in the coffin was returning home to a cold, empty house with no dinner on the bloody table. He opened the fridge, assuming that Fiona might have left a plate of something, but it seemed not. He glanced around the kitchen. The girl hadn't been back at all that day by the looks of things. Stuck consoling her friend, no doubt. God alone knew what women found to say to one another. Hours on end they could spend talking. He'd seen it with Fiona before. After forty-five minutes on the phone to her damn sister, he'd ask and she'd shrug.

'What?' he'd say. 'You're costing us a fortune in bills and you don't even know what it was you were talking about?'

That was so like Fiona though. She'd probably enjoyed the comforting arms of that damn gamekeeper Kenneth also. Gregory had no doubt that he would have been only too keen to offer his taxiing services that morning if it meant spending a few extra minutes with Fiona. Gregory wondered if the man really admired her, or if it was as much to irritate him as anything.

Gregory climbed the stairs still thinking of his wife. He'd

have a shower and then phone her. He supposed she would probably need picking up from Rosemary's house. He could do that and go in past for a chip supper on the way home.

He froze as he was removing his shirt, his arm halfway out of the sleeve. What if Rosemary decided, after all, to return with Fiona? Oh, God, how awful it would be. How awkward and embarrassing. How would he cope tiptoeing around the weeping woman? Of course, there was the question of who she would blame also. Gregory knew only too well that it would be him. Not just Rosemary, but bloody Adam Foster and Mr Dewhurst already thought he had been involved. When the police came knocking, he imagined that they would think the same. The unfairness of it all. His fist clenched involuntarily. He was done with self-pity, but instead, he found that deep within, it had been replaced by a wave of seething anger.

He thought back to his conversation with Adam that morning and the odious man's smug theory that Gregory had deliberately injured his guest. The very thought! He had enough on his plate without plotting elaborate ways to kill people, especially when they mattered so little to him as David Holden. What motive might he, Gregory, have had for bumping the idiot off? Gregory knew that Adam hadn't believed him when he denied it. Not that Adam could prove a thing. It was strange thinking back to that morning. It seemed a lifetime ago now. Adam and he had done a kind of dance, with first, one believing that they had the upper hand, and then the other. Both men despised one another, that was clear, but both knew, that to stay safe, they must protect the other.

'Mr Dewhurst seemed a bit cut up about it,' Gregory had said after the old man left.

Adam had nearly spat at him. 'Of course, he damn well is. We all are.'

Gregory snorted. 'You couldn't give a monkey's about the

dead man, it's your reputation that's of concern. Bloody false, that's what you are.'

Adam's face twisted. 'Can I remind you, that it was *your* gun? You're the one for it if it comes to anything. You should have checked the barrel was clear. He was your responsibility at the time. He was a novice. What are the police going to find when they look at the thing anyway? Did you tamper with it or not?'

Gregory shook his head. 'It was clean,' he said. 'I told you that already. I was about to shoot the damn thing myself. It was all David's idea. He pressed me to have a go. It could easily have been me lying there dead.'

Adam leaned back in his chair. 'And you think the police will believe that story? What was it then? Was he playing around with your missus? I've heard she's easily swayed but then who can blame her with you as her husband?'

Gregory pushed his chair back. It clattered sideways on the ground. His strong hands gripped the edge of Adam's desk and his jaw tightened. Gregory felt his temples pulsate.

'Sit down, you idiot,' Adam hissed and looked away.

'Say that again. Go on. Say it again, and I'll bloody have you. You're on borrowed time yourself, you jumped-up bastard. What would Mr Dewhurst say if he knew what I knew? What would he say if he realised his trusted estate manager was the real cause of his money worries?'

Adam had rolled his eyes. 'The place was a mess already. I've not caused that. Silly old man doesn't have a brain for business at all. Wouldn't know if he was being swindled by half a dozen people. All I did was redistribute a few of the salaries. It's not my fault he never checked the books.'

'As well as bumping up your own wages, you've been short-changing half the staff on the farm,' Gregory said.

'What, and you see yourself as some sort of crusader for the masses?' Adam scoffed. 'I hardly think so, Greg. You're only interested in yourself. We're no different from one another really when it comes down to it.'

Gregory shook his head remembering the conversation as he stepped into the shower. No, Adam was wrong. They weren't the same. But at least in Adam, he had an ally of sorts. A dangerous one, who he couldn't trust as far as he could throw him, but an aide all the same. By the end of their little chat, it was quite clear to Gregory, that the spineless fool didn't want to ruin a good thing. It seemed that Adam was already tied into paying a hefty mortgage and any shortfall now might ruin him. That's what had started him on the scheme in the first place he had said. Greed, Gregory thought to himself. It was indeed a dreadful thing.

The hot water drummed on Gregory's scalp and he closed his eyes. He hadn't confided in Adam of course. Who could he speak to though? He had so many suspicions. He'd not talk to Fiona, that was for sure. The girl's silly carry-on with Kenneth had obviously stirred the attentions of the farm staff. Who knew where her loyalties lay now? He had assumed that she had been quite honest with him about her association with the gamekeeper. Admittedly, he didn't like the alliance. Well, what man would like his young wife chattering away with the gamekeeper's type? Smarmy, that was what bloody Kenneth was. Smarmy and crawling. The way he had carried on at the fatal shoot, stepping into Adam's shoes and taking over. It made Gregory sick.

He turned off the shower and reached for the towel. As he rubbed furiously at his wet mop of hair he thought back to the day. Who had tampered with his gun? Someone must have. Was it Kenneth? At first, it seemed that just about anyone might have, but if he thought about it hard, few had had the opportunity. He had indeed left the case unattended. It was a foolish oversight on his part. But while the commotion at the river was ongoing, he knew for sure that both Adam Foster and most of the shooting party had been with him, not rummaging around in the boot of his Land Rover. Gregory forced himself to think hard. Fiona and Rosemary had been by the edge of the river. It was Fiona in fact, who had forced him into intervening. Adam and Mr Dewhurst had been present also. Even David himself, he had seen. Only Kenneth the bloody gamekeeper was left then. Could it possibly have been him?

Gregory thought, screwing up his eyes with the effort of it. Had he noticed where the greasy gamekeeper was during the chaos? He had been there over lunch. Gregory had spotted the creep talking to Fiona and Rosemary. They had been laughing away together.

Gregory pulled the towel from his head and began to dry his torso. He went through the events of that day in his mind, of passing David as he ran and then crashing out of the field gate and into the bramble bushes. He paused, the towel hovering over his chest. Of course, why had he been so stupid? Someone had been with him at the time. But who had it been? Gregory tried to remember a face. Someone had followed him. He had been trying to see the dog as it came downstream. Gregory had called for the other person in the bushes to pass him something with enough reach, that he might scoop out the dog as it drifted past.

Gregory allowed the towel to drop to the floor. But they hadn't passed him a stick, had they? He thought of himself teetering on the edge of the river. Instead of being handed a branch, the person behind him had done something else. Gregory shook his head in recollection. Of course. He had felt a firm hand on his back. Someone had deliberately pushed. Naturally, he had slipped and fallen in. Oh, how he wished now, that he had looked back and seen who it had been. Who had pushed him forcefully into the fast-flowing river, knowing that if a dog had drowned in it, he too might be swept away? Who, after failing to gain anything through this nasty plan, had instead crept back up to the field through the bushes whilst everyone's attention was on the river? Who had opened his gun case, knowing that he might well shoot that afternoon, and sabotaged the thing?

Gregory hastily wrapped the towel that had fallen to the ground around his waist and stumbled downstairs. On the bannister, hung his tweed jacket. With shaking hands, he felt for what he knew must still be there. He found it and, in the hallway, still damp from his shower and quite unaware of how cold it was becoming, Gregory studied his find. It had been on the ground beside David's body. Surely, it seemed all too clear that this had been the cause of the gun's misfire. Gregory turned it over in his damp fingers, feeling the rough, dented surface of the Roman coin. Who had placed this inside his gun barrel, knowing full-well that it would cause it to backfire? And given that he was the one who was meant to shoot it, who then had wanted him, Gregory, dead?

28

When Cathy arrived back at the surgery, she was restless and chilly. She stalked about her consultation room, knowing that she must call in her first patient but feeling too twitchy to do so. Shivering, she crossed to the radiator and turned the dial up to full, then telling herself that really, she had little choice and that James was counting on her to run a tight ship, she sat down at her desk and looked at her list of patients for the afternoon.

Having dispatched her first two simple cases quickly, Cathy rested back in her chair. She knew that something odd had happened to bring about the man's tragic death up at the farm. She realised that it sounded like an accident, but Mr Dewhurst's suspicion was concerning, and if the old man suspected Gregory of being involved, it seemed likely that the police might come to this conclusion also. Well, Cathy thought, that might not be such a bad thing. She had disliked the man on meeting him. She already had her uncertainties about how he treated his wife also. But how would this impact her? Would they ask why she signed off the licence?

Cathy glanced at her computer screen. Her next patient was

waiting. Before she called them through, she hesitated. What did Mr Dewhurst expect her to do? She had felt almost black-mailed into helping. She could hardly go bumbling in asking questions without provoking suspicion. She had already been indiscreet in doing an unnecessary home visit to the Warren-ders. Cathy thought of Fiona's male friend. Was the girl as inno-cent as she appeared? Cathy was quite convinced that she was up to her eyeballs in something unpleasant. But really, was it any of her business?

It was just after six when her final patient left. She was due at Suzalinna's house at seven-thirty for a well-overdue catch-up with her friend. Suzalinna had been leaving repeated answer-phone messages since they last spoke and the previous evening, after a large glass of wine, Cathy had finally agreed. She knew that she should really be typing up her revalidation paperwork, but there was always the weekend.

Cathy began to close down the computer. One of the locum doctors passed her door and then seeing her still seated at her desk, the man waved.

'Tomorrow we do it all again,' he called and she smiled.

The rest of the work could wait until the morning. She tidied her desk, moving her diagnostic set and slipping pens back into the holder by her prescription pad. Then, turning off the radi-ator behind her desk, she twisted in her chair to find Julie, one of the receptionists, at the door.

'Knock, knock,' the girl said and grinned.

'Oh, Julie. Come in. I was about to call it a day. Don't tell me there's something else?'

'Sorry to bother you, Dr Moreland. Yes, I saw everyone was packing up.'

Cathy was collecting her bag, glanced up and saw that Julie was still hovering in a distracted manner.

'Well, what is it?' she asked. She didn't have time for this really if she was to shower and get changed. She'd also need to pick up a bottle of wine to take to Suzalinna's house. She had planned to take the one in the cupboard, but given the stress over the past week, she'd somehow managed to finish it herself.

Julie came further into the room. 'I would have turned her away. I know it's after six and by rights, she should be seen by the out-of-hours doctors now, but it's the circumstances, you see?'

'Who? What circumstances, Julie? I'm hashed and wanting to get away. Don't play guessing games with me.'

Julie approached. 'She's in a bit of a state,' she hissed.

Cathy turned. 'What?'

Julie glanced behind. 'The woman. Weird-looking, she is. Seems like she's frightened.'

Cathy tutted. 'Who? I'm assuming she's one of ours?' She jabbed at the start button on her computer. The machine beeped twice and then whirred into action. 'Well?' she repeated.

'Young girl. Fiona Warrender. I know it's a pest. She seems so upset. Sort of exhausted. What could I say? I promised I would ask, but I warned her you might not be able to see her this evening.'

Cathy blinked slowly. Fiona Warrender had come to her? She shook her head in confusion and then smiled at her receptionist. 'Sorry, Julie. Show her through. I'll see her now.'

Julie looked relieved and scuttled away. Cathy sat back and waited, wondering just how she had become so entwined in this whole business.

29

Cathy did a double-take when she saw her. Julie had been correct in what she had said. Fiona Warrender did indeed look exhausted, but she had a frozen, almost haunted quality about her that Cathy had not expected. The woman smiled slightly and closing the door behind, sat down. Cathy studied her pale features, the hollowness of her cheeks and the almost-bruised skin around her eyes. There was no sign of emotion though. Strange. The last time they had met, despite being nervous, she had been so animated, so full of life.

'I'm sorry to do this,' she was saying. 'I realise now that you should have finished for the day. Time has been a little crooked for me. The girl at the front desk said she'd ask, but I didn't want to presume. I realise I've been a dreadful pest already to everyone.'

'Mrs Warrender, I'm glad to see you. I must admit that I've been a little concerned. I went out to your house today when I heard the news about the man's death this weekend. Your husband was involved in some way? His gun? I can see it's been a strain.'

The woman seemed to be focusing on something out of the

window. Cathy knew though that the sky was quite dark and she must see little other than her reflection in the glass.

'Oh, dear. I'm sorry. You drove all that way, did you?' she asked in a monotone, shaking her head slightly. 'I seem to have caused a good deal of bother.'

Cathy smiled. 'I felt I had a duty of care to check on you. When you last came in, you said things had been awkward at home. Fiona?'

The woman's eyelids fluttered. 'Well, not the best. This, obviously ... Well, it's changed things. I assume you heard all the details now about the accident up at the farm? It was my friend's husband that died. I've spent the day with her. Not great,' she said in answer to the unvoiced question. 'In shock, I suppose you'd call it. I've never seen Rosemary so detached. Upsetting really. I know she blames me, well us. She didn't actually accuse Gregory, but it's the only conclusion, isn't it? The way she looked at me. It was like she hardly knew me. It's unsurprising really.'

Cathy was confused. 'I can understand her being distraught, of course. In the early stages of grief, it's quite common to look to attribute blame. It may be that as time goes on, she'll soften. Things must be very raw.'

Fiona shook her head. 'No, you don't understand. Time won't make this better. It's ruined. Everything's ruined. I know it's the last time she'll speak to me. I know it.'

'If it was your husband's gun, I can see her reasoning in being angry initially, but you? Why would you be responsible, Fiona?'

'Well, I arranged it, didn't I? If it hadn't been for me insisting on having the Holdens over for a meal, David might never have been on the shoot.' Fiona twisted her hands in her lap. 'And then it was Gregory's gun. David had asked to use it, just as a one-off. He had one already, borrowed from the estate. They lend them out to guests who don't have their own. That afternoon though, for some reason, they swapped over. Gregory handed his own gun to David and well, you know the rest.'

'I heard it backfired.'

'Yes. It exploded in his face. I don't know anything about guns but they don't often backfire. Since the accident, things at home ...'

Cathy waited.

'Gregory. He's been odd. Well, I told you already that things were strained, but since the accident, it's been awful. It's like he simply won't communicate. He thinks I'm having an affair.' The girl looked up from her hands, her eyes meeting Cathy's for the first time and then dropping once more.

'And are you?'

Fiona smiled sadly.

'I don't know how I can help,' Cathy said rather desperately. It seemed to her that the conversation was going in circles.

Fiona Warrender inhaled deeply and shifted in her seat. When she looked up again, her eyes were dark and her voice was almost a whisper. 'I wonder about the gun,' she said.

'Yes?' Cathy asked.

The girl nodded. 'Yes. I do wonder about the gun. Oh, I don't know what I'm saying really. It's just, how could it have happened? Rosemary didn't come right out with it today, but I could see it was on her mind. Why David's dead and not Gregory? Well, it should have been my husband. It was his gun. What were the chances of him handing it to someone else to shoot?'

Cathy nodded. 'Yes. Well, if there was a mechanical issue with the gun, had Gregory mentioned it behaving strangely that morning when he was shooting? I'll be honest, I'm no expert in firearms.'

The girl shook her head. 'Oh no, I see what you mean. No, Gregory hadn't taken it out of the case at all that morning. He was supervising the shoot, overseeing the less experienced ones. He was allowed to take part, but only if the men he was looking after were deemed qualified enough to take care of themselves.'

'So, by lunchtime, he was sure?'

'Yes. I went out there, as it happens. We both did; me and Rosemary, to take the boys their lunch. I was glad to have her company. Gregory was in a dreadful mood. Spiteful. The things he was saying and in front of people too,' Fiona said. 'It was a relief to leave in the end. David promised he'd get him cheered up by the time they were done. I didn't want him coming back to the house, you see? I was frightened of him; he was so angry that day. I think David understood.'

Cathy nodded. 'Oh, dear. So, you and Rosemary went back to the house. Was that when you heard the news?'

Fiona grimaced. 'We heard the sirens as it happens and had a bit of a laugh about it. It seems utterly sickening to think of us sitting in my kitchen, joking about one of the toffs falling in the river when it was David lying dead in the field. Rosemary didn't stay long. She had things to do at home, so she left not long after. I assume the police went straight to her house and told her when the hospital confirmed it.'

Cathy sighed. 'I wonder what can have happened with the gun.'

'I heard most of the details from Kenny. He drove me to Rosemary's this morning. Gamekeeper,' Fiona said and blushed.

Fiona was certainly playing a dangerous game if she was having an affair.

'Gregory wouldn't tell me much himself, but he did say that David had borrowed the gun. He'd not used it at all himself, so he said. David shot it for the first time and that's when it backfired.'

'I see. It's a bit of a mystery then. But no doubt the estate will get to the bottom of it though. The police will examine the gun, I assume?'

Fiona's eyes grew wide. She clasped her hands tightly in her lap. 'I suppose they will. Oh God, but what will they find? What if it was Greg's fault?' The girl went to pieces completely, sobbing uncontrollably. 'I'm in deep water already, quite apart from all of this. Gregory and I are in a real mess. I think you knew that from when I was last in. I thought he was trying to kill me. Poison! Perhaps I was right in what I said. I do wonder. He's filled with anger sometimes. He didn't like David; I do know that. Called him stuck-up. He never has liked people who he feels are superior. What if he is to blame? What then? What if Gregory did do it?'

'Well the police need to find out the truth,' Cathy said. 'A man has died. They must find answers, not only for his widow but if it was an accident so that it can be prevented from happening again.'

The girl seemed not to listen. 'There's an odd atmosphere,' she was saying. 'I've been out all day because of it. Oh, I needed to see Rosemary, of course. I tried to get her to come back with me, but what would I be bringing her into? I'm almost afraid to go back to the house now myself. It's cursed or something. I wanted to move. He'll never allow it though. I'm deathly afraid, Dr Moreland. Deathly afraid.' The girl turned sheet-white.

Cathy was speechless. It did cross her mind that Fiona Warrender might be suffering from some kind of persecution complex given what she had just said. It wasn't the first time she had spoken sensationally about her fears. Was her suggestion earlier of her husband poisoning her, simply a symptom? A paranoid delusion or an over-valued idea? Cathy began to wonder as she watched the young girl attempt to gain control of her emotions. She passed the box of tissues across the desk.

Fiona dabbed at her eyes and blew her nose noisily. 'I'm

making a dreadful fool of myself; I know. You probably think I'm crazy.'

Cathy smiled at the aptness of the woman's words. 'Well,' she said. 'I'd not put it that way, but you are distressed. Have you had any other worrying thoughts? Any unusual ideas?'

The girl laughed harshly. 'Oh, so you do think that. I came here for help, not to be locked away in a mental home. I'm not mad. But I *am* afraid. I chose you. I'd heard about you.'

'Mrs Warrender, I have a duty of care to my patients ...'

'Well, I'm your patient! Don't I matter? As a doctor, you're meant to be dependable, full of principle.' The girl's eyes were wild with anger and a few droplets of saliva landed on the desk. 'I trusted you when we first met. But now I'm frightened. Really frightened. What if the police think this wasn't an accident? What if they think Gregory was involved? What if you send me home tonight and I'm sleeping beside a murderer?'

30

Rosemary's mother arrived in Glainkirk on Wednesday afternoon. When Rosemary saw her getting out of the taxi, she felt an almost childlike relief wash over her. But her mother's black dress and grave countenance gave a sharp reminder of the harsh reality of the situation.

She had slept little the previous night. This wasn't so unexpected. She had thought about taking one of David's tablets. He had been prescribed them months back when he was struggling to relax. It had been when he was trying to do some big deal or other for the agents and then he ended up pulling a muscle in his back or neck. He had become so pumped up about the thing that he couldn't calm down at bedtime. Rosemary had found herself the previous evening in the bathroom, standing at the sink with the packet of pills in her hand. They were probably out of date by now and next to useless. She held the packet for some time wondering what in the world this life held for her now.

Her mother's cheek was wrinkled and cold when she pressed her own to it. Nothing had changed between them. Rosemary had hoped that the older woman might have thawed somewhat, but apparently not.

'Dreadful business,' her mother said.

'I thought Dad might ...'

'He's busy with work,' her mother answered and pursed her lips.

Rosemary carried her mother's bag through and placed it at the bottom of the stairs. She watched the older woman take the place in, looking up and down the hallway and glancing into the dining room.

'Of course, you've not seen the new house,' Rosemary said. 'I'll show you up to your room in a minute. I'm glad you came, thank you. It's been a difficult couple of days.'

Her mother nodded. 'I assume the police ...'

'Oh yes. Quite sympathetic. I suppose they're used to, well ...' Rosemary tailed off seeing her mother's look of incredulity.

'Hardly,' her mother said. 'I doubt they're used to anything of the kind, Rosemary. I should think there's been a postmortem?'

Rosemary gulped.

'Well? I should think so. What have they said so far? Someone must be liable.'

'The gun ... The estate he was shooting with, they lent out ...'

'Well then. They must have insurance. Someone will be to blame. You don't want to hear it now, but you'll be due compensation of some sort. You can't live on fresh air for the rest of your life, Rosemary.'

'I have a job.'

Her mother laughed. 'Yes, well, as I say, you can't live on fresh air.'

'I'll put the kettle on, shall I?' she asked. 'The journey up, how was it?'

Her mother was moving around the living room. She paused at the mantlepiece.

Oh God, don't touch his photo.

But the old woman had already lifted the one of David when they had been on holiday in the south of France the previous year. He had a glass of wine in his hand and was smiling at her, the photographer. She wanted to cross the room and snatch the picture from her mother, but instead, she stood in the doorway and clenched her teeth.

'It's always very cold up in Scotland, isn't it? No doubt a sunnier climate would have been a relief.'

Her mother put the photograph back down and moved along the line of condolence cards, picking up one or two and smiling at the words.

Rosemary nodded and went through to the kitchen, unable to watch any longer.

It had been such a long time; she had almost forgotten why she rarely saw her mother. David had outright hated the woman. He called her a 'frosty, old bitch.' Rosemary had scolded him for it several times over the years, but in the current circumstances, she found herself smiling in fondness at the shared joke.

When the tea was made, Rosemary found her mother seated on one of the armchairs in the cool sunshine.

'You look tired,' the old woman accused. 'and a little irritable too.'

'The funeral directors are coming later, I think.'

Her mother tutted. 'I'd forget about that for now. Oh, choose your hymns or whatever you're planning by all means.'

'Mum, why are you being so ...?'

'Why am I being so what, Rosemary? Realistic? You know I'll not lie to you. I never have. I disliked David, but I wouldn't wish widowhood on you for a minute. Certainly not at your age. Mind you, I suppose you'll at least have a chance to meet someone else in the years to come. Possibly, it was all meant to be. Perhaps you'll choose more wisely the second time around.'

Rosemary gripped the edge of the chair.

Her mother observed her. Her eyes had a spirited look about them.

'I do think you have to be honest, Rosemary. At the very least, with yourself,' the old woman continued. 'This might be the making of you. But let's not beat about the bush. If the police are involved and a postmortem is in progress, there won't be a funeral. Not for some time to come. I have no idea how the legal system works up here. An inquest, or something of the kind, will have to take place.'

Rosemary exhaled. Despite her tactlessness, perhaps her mother was right. She had no idea how it would work out. She had hoped that the funeral arrangements and the event itself, might act as a kind of distraction from the odd in-between state in which she currently found herself. She was quite sure that the police had explained this to her at the start. The liaison officer had sat with her for some time. She had been in no position to take anything in though. It was normal, she supposed; to feel this odd numbness. It was the shock of the thing. People had said that to her, but she had no idea how they knew. Did anyone know how it felt?

The days since David's death had passed in something of a haze. She thought of Fiona's visit the other day, when they had sat and drunk tea and Rosemary hadn't heard a word the other girl said. Fiona had prattled on and on about how awful it all was. At the time, Rosemary wasn't sure how she felt about Fiona coming. She was her friend, of course, so it was only natural that she should want to be supportive. But the more Rosemary had considered things, especially during her last wakeful night, the more she thought that she'd rather not see Fiona again. No, she'd be quite content never to set eyes on her ever again. It seemed strange to feel the friendship change so suddenly as if a switch had been flicked. What on earth did they now have in common anyway? Maybe it wasn't Fiona at all, maybe it was her husband.

Rosemary felt herself go cold. Her mother was saying something in an austere, logical sort of voice, but she couldn't bring herself to listen. She thought of Gregory Warrender and his blotched face during dinner that night when they had been invited over. She thought of his stupid, drunken bravado and his fat fist as he thumped the table to further some point he had been making. Rosemary knew only too well that Fiona wished it was he who had died. She could see it in the way the girl spoke. She didn't blame her.

Suddenly, Rosemary found herself thinking of the old woman on the train. She had warned Rosemary and said that Fiona should take care. And how right she had been. Gregory was indeed an odious creature. For some months, Rosemary had suspected that Fiona was growing more anxious about her husband. And, of course, it turned out to have been Gregory's gun that had killed David. Rosemary hoped with every ounce of her being that the horrible man would pay for his mistake.

31

'Well darling, I don't know what to make of it,' Suzalinna said, resting back on the rattan chair and folding her bare feet under her.

'Bit odd isn't it?' Cathy agreed.

They were sitting together in Suzalinna's conservatory. Saj had just refilled their glasses and then excused himself saying that he had paperwork to do. Cathy had grinned up at him and he had winked knowingly.

Now, in the candlelight, Cathy smiled across at her old medical-school comrade. How glad she was of the friendship but how dreadful she had been at keeping in touch these past few months. It hadn't taken long for Cathy to explain her strange consultation with Fiona Warrender, and her unusually strong dislike towards the young woman's husband. She had begun to run through the events since David Holden's death too, with Suzalinna interrupting only occasionally to clarify a point.

'I thought it was a straight-forward enough thing, though,' Suzalinna said. 'Admittedly, Mr Holden's death was a tragedy, but surely it had to be a silly accident. When I referred the case to the police, I didn't think it was murder.'

'That's what I assumed too, although the girl, Fiona, and her husband have given me several sleepless nights this last week.'

Suzalinna looked puzzled and Cathy sighed.

'Oh, well it's all rather odd. Fiona came in to see me first. She had some silly complaint about dry skin and her hair falling out. I did a blood test to check the obvious stuff, you can imagine, but there were a couple of things during the consultation that worried me.'

Suzalinna raised her eyebrows but didn't speak.

'So, the first thing was her story,' Cathy said. 'She said that the dry skin had been going on for a few weeks. Went into detail about how she was having to cover her blotches up with thick make-up. She's quite like that; dolled up, and I don't want to say superficial, but you know what I mean? She seemed embarrassed to admit her real concern, but when she did finally come out with it, she told me she had wondered if her husband was trying to kill her.'

'What?' Suzalinna laughed and in doing so, almost spilt her glass of wine.

Cathy smiled. 'I know. It does sound ludicrous, doesn't it? But after all of this week's business, I'm now beginning to wonder. So, she thought he was poisoning her. When she voiced it, she actually started back-tracking and telling me she'd been watching too many horrors on TV, but the suggestion made me rather suspicious. At the time, I was less concerned about that and more about the bruise on her arm.'

'Oh, I see,' Suzalinna said, meaningfully. She paused and sipped her wine. 'You think the husband? Perhaps he wasn't poisoning her, but mistreating her in some way?'

Cathy grimaced. 'I'm really not sure now. It all seems a bit fanciful. She was edgy. You know how these people are when they come in? It gave me a kind of sick feeling that I was missing something though, even at the time before all this shooting nonsense kicked off. But I wasn't a hundred per cent sure. If I had been, I might have confronted her, but I would have hated doing that too.' Cathy sighed. 'She certainly didn't confide in me that much, but when I asked about her menstrual cycle ...'

'Thyroid?'

'Yes, I did wonder about hypothyroidism. I checked for TFTs when I took her blood. It came back normal, by the way. All of her bloods were fine. But, like I was saying, when I asked about her periods, she went all defensive and thought I was accusing her of being pregnant.'

'Accusing? But what would have been wrong with her being pregnant?'

'Well, exactly. It did make me wonder if something else was going on. I met the husband by chance the following week. He was in getting his gun licence renewed. I hate doing the bloody things, but there seemed no reason not to sign. He had no mental health issues, no drug or alcohol misuse in his history. I only realised who he was halfway through the consultation, as it happens. I wavered a bit when I knew. It was just following what his wife had said. But I couldn't not sign, if you see what I mean? Now, I'm wondering, given that it was his gun that actually killed the man, should I have done it?'

'Oh God Cathy,' Suzalinna said.

Cathy looked imploringly at her friend. 'What was I to do though, Suz? I had no reason not to sign.'

Suzalinna nodded but didn't speak.

'Listen, I even drove up to the cottage to check on her after I heard about the shooting accident. That's how careful I was being,' Cathy argued. 'I didn't like the husband at all when he came in. He wasn't threatening, but I felt I had been manipulated in some way. I don't think he's a nice person, but I can't penalise someone for that. I checked with the reception girls and he paid the fee for the paperwork without question. Didn't mess them around at all.'

'I know you're saying all this,' Suzalinna said. 'And it sounds fine.' She paused and Cathy wondered what her friend was going to say. 'Well, you clearly don't believe it yourself, do you? You say it was fine, that you had no choice signing the form. That I agree with. But you then felt the need to drive to their house ... Well, it speaks volumes doesn't it?'

Cathy exhaled. 'I suppose it does. I was worried. And I didn't even manage to see her. I did, however, meet someone else. The gamekeeper.'

Suzalinna grinned.

'Oh yes, you'd have liked him,' Cathy said laughing. 'He seemed to know a lot about the couple and especially the wife. Very handsome, curly hair, a bit rough and ready.'

'Sounds right up my street,' Suzalinna snorted.

'Poor Saj,' Cathy scolded. 'I doubt that a husband would take kindly to him hanging around, especially Fiona's brute of a man.'

'Do you think she's having an affair then?'

'I don't know. Maybe. Probably. But it still leaves me in a mess.'

Suzalinna put her glass of wine down and stared intently at her friend. 'Tell me properly what she said this last time then when she came in today.'

'Well, it was all so dramatic,' Cathy said. 'She was in tears for a good bit of the consultation. I'm still unclear as to how she thinks I can help.'

'Does she need your help though? Is it even a medical issue?'

Cathy sighed. 'She was histrionic to the extreme. Said that she was scared of going back to the house. I did wonder if she was actually delusional. If I hadn't already met her husband, I might well have believed she was mentally unwell. She seems to have convinced herself that this man's death wasn't a mistake, or at the very least, she thinks that the police will discover something was wrong about the whole thing. David was using her husband's gun,' Cathy explained. 'Her husband hadn't shot at all that day, but for some reason, he handed his gun to this man, David. He stood beside him as he shot the thing, and you know how that ended.'

Suzalinna whistled. 'So, she thinks that her husband did something to make the gun backfire in David's face? I don't know how you'd even go about doing something like that. Stuff something down the barrel, I suppose? Seems a bit crude, doesn't it?'

Cathy shrugged. 'I hate guns and I don't know the first thing about them, but that's what she intimated anyway.'

'So, how have you left it then? Is she coming back to see you?'

'She was quite angry in the end when I said I was reluctant to get involved.'

'Surely the police will be looking into it though,' Suzalinna said settling back on the cushions.

'Well, of course, I did say that, but she's not the only person to approach me ...'

Suzalinna looked quizzical.

'Yes. Old Mr Dewhurst who owns the estate. He's been a patient of ours for a long time. James usually deals with him, but what with him being away, I've taken over. I went out last week as it happens. In fact, he didn't really warrant a house call and I think James has been coerced into it. I told him he needed to come into the surgery from now on. I don't think he liked that too much. Anyway,' Cathy said, seeing that she was going off track. 'He phoned me. It was before Fiona came in. He told me that he wanted someone sensitive to look into the case.'

Suzalinna guffawed. 'Your reputation precedes you, darling!'

Cathy swatted her friend. 'Oh don't. I knew you'd laugh. This time, I must say I'm disinclined to get involved. I'm up to here with work, keeping on top of the locums. Just this afternoon, I caught one of them almost getting us sued for negligence. He'd been dictating his referrals all week, not realising that he had them stacked up, needing to be signed before their dispatch. Two of them were urgent ones. I signed them myself and caught up with him only later on to say. It scares me that people can be so lax. The buck stops with me, after all. If things aren't done correctly, I'll get it. He'll move onto his next job in a couple of weeks and I'll be left picking up the pieces.'

'When is James back?'

Cathy smiled. 'Not for another week. I promised him, you see? I wanted everything in good order. I wanted to prove to him I was capable. It's been so long since he's trusted me to be in charge for more than a few days. I wanted to show him that he was right. That I can do it.'

Suzalinna smiled. 'Yes. I did wonder. Well, perhaps that's your answer then. You're worrying about whether you should get involved in this thing, but in the same sentence, you've told me, you're too stressed. Cathy darling, you can't save everyone. And really, you shouldn't have to. The police have their responsibilities and you have yours. Your job description did not encompass getting involved in strange deaths, the last time I looked. I think you've had more than your fair share of adventures recently.'

Cathy nodded. Of course, her friend was right, the duties of a doctor did not include unravelling mysteries, but they did consist of taking prompt action if she felt a patient was at risk. Cathy wondered if she could let the thing go, knowing that Fiona Warrender might be in danger. She sipped her wine meditatively in silence and the conversation moved on. But by the end of the evening, as she kissed Suzalinna and Saj good-night, she had already decided that she could not leave it. Mr Dewhurst's ambiguous threat still rang in her ears. No, in the morning, she would go to work early. She'd get her lab results checked and her paperwork done, freeing up time later. If Fiona Warrender's suspicions were correct, Cathy would never forgive herself for not trying to help. She'd never forgive herself if she failed to prevent a further tragedy.

32

Cathy did indeed arrive early, having slept little the previous night. She was first into the practice and found that even the low buzz of the overhead electric lighting acted as an irritation. She found herself repeatedly glancing out at the car park as her thoughts drifted back to the fatal shooting and the Warrenders. But by eight o'clock, she had seen to her blood results, categorizing them according to what action should be taken.

Cathy was checking her emails when she heard the back-door bang and then footsteps sounded in the carpeted corridor. She had left her consulting room door ajar, and Michelle, her lead receptionist passed and then came back, seeing Cathy look up from her notes.

'Morning Dr Moreland,' the young woman said. 'You're in early today, aren't you?'

Cathy leaned back in her chair and stretched. 'Morning. Yes, I wanted to get a head start today. How are you? I think we've still got appointments, by the looks of things, but who knows how long it will last.'

Michelle smiled knowingly. 'I'll try to keep them from bothering you if I can.' The girl then came further into the room. 'I wondered if you'd heard any more about the shooting?' she asked. 'Julie said Mrs Warrender had been in yesterday in a bit of a state.'

Cathy looked at the girl.

'Oh, I don't want to know any medical details,' Michelle said hurriedly. 'I just wondered; you see? There's been a good bit of talk.'

'Oh? What kind of talk?'

'Gossip, I suppose really,' Michelle admitted. 'Around the town, folk have been saying things, and when they've been in here too. The man who died wasn't even our patient, but you can imagine how people like to go on when it's something unusual. I did hear that the police weren't happy.'

'Well, you know more than me then. I hadn't heard that at all. How do you know?'

Michelle smiled. 'Bert's son-in-law.'

Cathy nodded. She had forgotten that the handyman for the practice, Bert, had a police connection. 'I see. Well, if you're after more news from me, there isn't any. I think Fiona Warrender's husband will be questioned undoubtedly as he was at the same shoot. It's a worrying time for Mrs Warrender as you might imagine. She had every right to come in to talk. That's what we're here for, although there's probably very little I can do, other than listen.'

Michelle nodded and began to inch towards the door.

'When you say the police aren't happy, Michelle ...'

The young girl nodded and smiled. 'The shotgun,' she said. 'Not happy with the way it looks, apparently. I don't know the details, of course, but Bert said that his son-in-law told him that the gun looked like it had been tampered with!'

The young receptionist stepped back a little, having delivered her final proclamation with suitable enthusiasm.

Cathy swallowed but didn't speak.

'Well, exactly,' Michelle said enthusiastically. 'Sounds like a bit of a mess, doesn't it? They're saying that the gun didn't belong to the man who died at all. It was Mr Warrender's. Well, you can imagine the implication.'

Cathy raised her eyebrows. 'What?' But with a dreadful, sinking feeling, she knew only too well what Michelle was going to say.

'Well, apparently there had been some bother between the two men, that's what they're saying. They say that Mr Warrender arranged the whole thing. He deliberately didn't shoot all that morning himself, because he'd doctored his gun ready to go off in the other man's face. They say Mr Warrender killed him and it was murder! What do you think of that?'

Cathy didn't answer. Although the suggestion came as no surprise, she still felt quite sick.

She continued her morning surgery, being as precise, discreet and friendly as she could manage. Beneath her shell of professionalism, however, she was profoundly uneasy. She knew how rapidly rumours spread. If the people of Glainkirk were now speculating as to the potential culprit, and Gregory had been named, it seemed impossible for him and his wife to escape the dreadful business unscathed. Cathy already had her concerns about Fiona Warrender's mental health. This gossip might well prove to be the breaking point for the delicate young woman.

When she was finished for the morning, Cathy closed her consulting-room door and leaned back heavily on the cool wood. She was disturbed by the town's folk's conclusion that Gregory was guilty. Why had they jumped to this deduction so readily? It didn't look good. Cathy knew only too well the phrase 'no smoke without fire.' She could only imagine how things might have escalated on the farm estate. Even Mr Dewhurst had been suspicious. Cathy had disliked Gregory when she met him also, but she did feel that they were getting rather a head of themselves. She had already begun to consider several other possibilities herself.

Firstly, one had to think of the man David Holden. If looking at the thing rationally, his death might fall into three possible categories: accident, suicide or murder. From what Michelle had told her, it now seemed that accidental death was unlikely if the police had indeed examined the gun and found something suspicious about the mechanism. That still didn't rule out suicide, but she had discounted the idea almost from the off, as there were surely far more reliable and rapid methods to kill one's self than chancing a gun's backfire. The process, after all, might easily have maimed only, leaving David burned and disfigured for the rest of his life. Cathy wished that she knew more about David Holden. It was so difficult to consider all of these theories without putting a face to the name.

Sighing, she crossed her room and stood by the window. The surgery car park backed onto school playing fields, and a group of teenagers wearing their own interpretation of the uniform passed by giggling. Cathy glanced at the clock on her wall. It was nearly her lunchtime too, not that she felt she could face anything to eat. Impulsively, she sat down at her computer once more and typed the name: 'Holden'. She knew that David wasn't registered with their practice, but he was a Glainkirk resident, and might conceivably have a family. Cathy already knew that he had a wife. Fiona Warrender had been to visit her before attending the surgery, she had said. Was it possible that she was a patient, even though her husband had failed to join?

There were four Holdens registered with the surgery. Two, Cathy could discount immediately, as they were in their eighties and resided at one of the nursing homes that she looked after. This left two others: Jessica Ann Holden, aged twenty-five, who might fit the bill, and Rosemary Holden, aged thirty-one. Both were potentials. Odd though, that if the widow was one of her patients, she hadn't been in touch.

Cathy quickly scanned through the first woman's notes. A regular attendee to the practice due to asthma. Linda, their salaried GP, had seen her for a routine chronic illness check a month or so ago, but otherwise, she was seen by the practice nurses to check her peak flows and her inhaler technique. They had given her the flu jab the last time also. Well, there was no mention of being married in the notes, unfortunately, but Cathy might ask if Linda knew the girl, or remembered anything about her. Then, she came to the other woman. Rosemary. It seemed that she had only joined the practice two years before. She had undergone the usual medical when registering but otherwise there was nothing. Cathy saw that the nurse dealing with her at the time had typed: 'Personal assistant, Greysons.' A memory stirred in Cathy's mind. She fought with herself trying to remember but it wouldn't come. No doubt it would occur to her if she let it alone. Well, either of these women might conceivably be related to Mr Holden, but it got her little further forward she supposed.

Still, it might be worthwhile pursuing. If David Holden had been deliberately killed, there really must be a strong motive. Admittedly, the most obvious person to tamper with the gun still seemed to be Gregory Warrender, but wasn't the most likely person to commit a murder usually the spouse? With her heart pounding at the thought, Cathy decided that she must certainly look into it.

33

Gregory leaned against the cold metal bar that surrounded the cattle court. His favourite cow had just delivered a bull-calf and it was taking a while to latch-on. He knew that the mother was experienced enough to deal with it, but he would stay to make sure. He watched the calf struggle to its feet, still slick, its brown and white coat shiny and matted. The mother, exhausted but attentive, leaned in and nuzzled her newborn.

'Proud of him, are you?' Gregory asked. 'You did fine.'

He sighed. Oh God, if he hadn't had this, where would he be? There was nothing for him at home. Fiona had been so strange and jumpy since the dreadful incident on the shoot. It was like she couldn't bear to be in his presence. She blamed him, he supposed, just like the rest of them. He'd heard the low snigger when he approached and then, when he was stood amongst the other farm lads, the conversation seemed stilted and odd. Yes, they were all avoiding him.

He watched as the calf faltered, but the mother, patient and stoic, nudged the thing closer to her belly. He heard the suckling noise and smiled to himself. Yes, thank God he could find some peace here, with his cattle. Gregory turned from the shed, and slowly crossed the dirt court to his jeep. He'd be back in later to check the calf had a full belly. He'd have come anyway, even if there wasn't a reason. His day ahead, after all, looked bleak.

That morning he had received a telephone call from Adam saying that the police would be visiting the estate office between half-past eleven and twelve. Gregory had been requested to attend for an 'informal interview'. To be honest, it came as little surprise. He was shocked that the police hadn't spoken to him earlier. It had been his gun after all and even if it had been a simple accident, he might be held as much to blame as anyone. But, of course, Gregory knew that it had not been an accident. He reached into his jacket pocket and turned the metal over in his hand. He had thought a good deal about whether he should tell the police about his discovery at the scene of the crime. Part of him wanted to blurt it out immediately so that it might clear his name. Why, at the end of the day, would he be stupid enough to show them the thing if he had himself rammed it down the gun barrel? But Gregory felt it best to keep his cards close to his chest. He had been thinking about the thing overnight and wondering who might have put it there. By choosing this object, rather than another one, such as a blank cartridge, he wondered if the killer was making some kind of a nasty point. If he himself was the intended victim, did it narrow the field?

Gregory had never been the best at problem-solving tasks, and even thinking about the thing made his head ache. He touched his brow and his forehead felt clammy. Perhaps he was actually coming down with something. He hoped not. He had no time for illness. There were still nine cows left to calve. He thought one of them might go tonight. She tended to be a tricky one. Fine, sturdy calves, but an unpredictable mother. No, but he must keep a clear head and his wits about him today of all days. If he saw any of the other farm lads, he'd give them a wide berth.

It didn't pass his attention that the police interviews were taking place in Adam Foster's office. No doubt it was more convenient for them to talk to all the estate staff there rather than tracking them to their individual homes, but how might anyone speak in confidence, knowing that they were on Mr Dewhurst's property? Gregory wasn't being paranoid, but he did wonder if the old man might listen in, or get his flunky Adam Foster to do so for him.

Things between him and Adam had been decidedly strained since their last meeting. Gregory had seen the estate manager about the farm and the pair had noticeably avoided one another. Even one of the farm lads had commented. Gregory had shrugged off the suggestion and told the boy that he and Adam had had a spat. It wasn't such an untruth anyway. Despite their common understanding, Gregory didn't trust the man as far as he could throw him.

Gregory went about his farm duties that morning with a morose certainty that something dreadful was about to happen. As he drove up to the cattle court nearing eleven, to check on the bull-calf before his appointment, he saw several cars already parked outside Adam's office. Well, Adam had said eleven-thirty, so he wasn't going to be earlier than that. He had already passed Potter's Field when he was delivering more strainer posts for the fence. He'd seen two people walking about the land, pointing and talking. They had been too far away to see properly, but Gregory thought that one of them had been Mr Dewhurst. Now that he'd thought about it, it seemed likely that the other had been a police officer. It was natural that the police might request a tour of the scene of the crime and the surrounding area. Gregory had watched police dramas on the television. He had thought that if they suspected a murder, they'd have been in white, hooded overalls, crawling about the grass looking for clues, but perhaps that was all a lot of nonsense.

As it turned out, the police inspector was smooth in his manner. He was almost coaxing in his way of talking and Gregory was reminded of how Adam Foster spoke to his gundogs when they refused to drop a dead bird. The policeman thanked Adam and dismissed him from the office. He then apologised for putting Gregory to the trouble of coming in when he was clearly so busy on the farm. He asked a little about the cattle they had and seemed knowledgeable on the subject. Gregory rather liked this and he felt himself swell with pride when he confided that his favourite had just calved that morning.

'A bull,' he said and the inspector nodded and smiled.

'For a beef farmer, that's the best outcome.'

'It is. We've a large enough herd as it is without more heifers,' Gregory said. 'Bulls are what make the money really.'

'Calf easily?' the inspector asked.

Gregory nodded. 'Good stock. Not too large. Most do it without the jack. She's known for it. Couthy, most of them.'

The inspector nodded. 'Partly breeding, but also the way they're handled. The more time you spend, the nicer natured they become.'

'Gentle hands, that's all they need,' Gregory said, enjoying the interview far more than he had anticipated. 'These young lads hurry too much. The cows don't appreciate that. Get narky and kick out. If you take your time, you get far better results in the end.'

The inspector smiled. 'Well, you're doing a grand job then. Now, I suppose I'd better ask some questions,' he laughed.

Gregory smiled and nodded again.

The questions were all rather obvious. First, the inspector wanted to know if Gregory could tell him anything about David Holden. Gregory described the man with impartiality he thought, although it was hard to refrain from displaying his disappointment at the other man's lack of skills when it came to handling a gun, especially given that he had boasted of his prowess only night before. When asked about his character, Gregory admitted that he knew him only superficially, but that he judged David to be a bit arrogant and full of hot air. He was asked to give details. Gregory blushed and admitted that he'd only really spoken with him at length once and it was just an impression. The policeman smiled disarmingly and Gregory confessed that on the occasion that David and his wife had come to have tea with them, he had found himself rather incapacitated. Something dodgy about the bottle of wine, he thought. The inspector grinned and agreed that he'd have a beer any day over some fancy wine. The two men laughed and the mood lightened a good deal.

The inspector went on to ask about the day of the shoot itself and how Gregory had arranged for his acquaintance to attend at the last minute. Gregory smirked and explained that he had been working there long enough to warrant the odd favour when it came to these matters. Finally, he was asked to go through the events of that day. This took some cajoling from the Inspector, as Gregory's recollection was slightly jumbled in its order of running, but eventually, they got there and Gregory leaned back in his chair and sighed.

'A nasty business,' the inspector admitted, placing his pen down after jotting a few notes. 'I wonder if you have a theory as to how it happened, yourself, Mr Warrender?'

Gregory wondered if the inspector asked this with a sharpness to his eye, but the man had spoken with the same casual, genial manner and he found himself relaxing.

'David wasn't my sort at all,' he confessed. 'He lived in a different world. He was more in the circle of the likes of our estate manager, or even Mr Dewhurst. What I did see of him, I didn't much like. I'm not fond of ambition when it means stamping on those below you, and I got the idea that David had few scruples when it came to that. He'd been wanting to come up here and shoot for a while, so it seems. At the time, I didn't know why, but I thought it would have been due to some scheme or other. Moving up the social ladder, or what have you. Now it seems I was partly right. He had designs on the land, Mr Dewhurst said. As for his death, I can't imagine how it happened. I know it was my gun, but it was clean, that I can tell you. Careful always, I was.'

The inspector nodded. 'Just so. Well, we did, as you might imagine, send the shotgun to the lab. It's pretty much regular procedure when it comes to this sort of an accident. Stops something else similar happening in the future hopefully and gives us answers as to why.'

Gregory held his breath.

The inspector shook his head and shifted his large frame as if he was adjusting himself for great mental concentration. 'It's a damn odd business, Mr Warrender, that I don't mind telling you. I hardly know what to say. Odd, it is. Damn odd. The lab came back with their usual complicated waffle. I'm too old to be learning all the ins and outs of technical jargon,' he said.

Gregory felt his stomach heave. The inspector's countenance had changed a good deal during the interview and his eyes were remarkably piercing.

'One thing came out of it though. Something that even I understood.'

The inspector chuckled to himself but Gregory didn't smile.

'The barrel of the gun, your shotgun, had some irregular scratches inside.'

The inspector paused. The room was silent bar the ticking of Adam Foster's clock.

'It seems likely that something was forced into the barrel. This blockage, one can only assume, caused the thing to back-fire in the unfortunate man's face. A devilishly odd affair, all in all. We'll have to investigate in detail, of course. I wonder if you could help us further, Mr Warrender? Perhaps down at the station? No, not to worry about letting them know, I've already spoken to Mr Foster and he's well aware where you'll be this afternoon. Better to get things cleared up, I always think, don't you?'

34

The house was set back from the road, and due to the slope of the hill on which it was positioned, the front door was reached by a steep flight of stone steps. Cathy adjusted her doctors' bag in her hand and began the ascent, using the handrail for support. Tricky with a bag of groceries, she thought to herself, and what if they had a child? Getting a pram up would be a nightmare. She then had the sickening realisation that if they did have a child, it would now be fatherless. Trying not to let her imagination run away with her, she jogged the last couple of steps and stood breathless at the top.

She had spoken to Linda before heading out. Unfortunately, her salaried colleague couldn't recall anything about Jessica Ann Holden. Cathy wasn't surprised. After all, why should she, unless the girl had said something really remarkable during the consultation? The GPs saw on average thirty patients a day. Remembering one from another, especially when doing a simple review, was impossible.

She knocked and then stepped back to wait. Of course, knowing her luck, the woman wouldn't even be at home and it would be a wasted journey. She turned from the door and looked out from her now elevated position across the street to the line of houses opposite and behind them, the smattering of town leading to open countryside. It made quite a view. Even in winter, the patchwork of fields was breathtaking. Cathy hastily turned, hearing a noise from behind and as she did so, the door was opened. The young woman looked a trifle dishevelled.

'Can I help?'

Cathy smiled. 'I'm sorry to disturb you,' she said, only then noticing the woman's night attire. 'I'm Dr Moreland from the Glainkirk Practice. I wondered if I might have a quick word?'

The woman seemed unsure. 'If it's about the prednisolone ...' she began, but Cathy shook her head and smiled.

'It's probably a bad time, but can I?'

The girl stepped back. 'I suppose so. I'm on nights, but that's me awake now.'

Cathy grimaced. 'Sorry. I suspect, if you're at work just now, I may well have woken you unnecessarily.'

As it turned out, she didn't need to stay for long to establish that this Ms Holden was not the one she was after. It was a rather awkward interview and Cathy was glad to leave. She thanked the woman for her time and hastily retreated to her car. Stupid to go crashing in bothering people. And the widow of Mr Holden might not even be on their patient register at all. Cathy checked the clock in her car. The other address wasn't more than five minutes from where she was now. She weighed up the embarrassment of knocking on another stranger's door, with finding the answer to her questions. It would probably be a waste of time but if she was quick, she'd make it back for afternoon surgery.

Cathy turned the car and signalled out onto the main street once more. The day was brightening and the hint at what spring might look like in a couple of months gave her some sign of hope. The street in which the second woman lived was wide and more ostentatious than the previous. In the driveways, Cathy saw several expensive cars. She came to the number she was after and saw in the window some flowers which, she thought might conceivably be a sign that she was on the right track. Of course, the woman might have bought herself the flowers, or her very much alive husband might have gifted them. But it could also be that they were a condolence gift. Cathy smiled slightly, realising that she was clutching at straws now.

The door was answered almost immediately. The woman's face was pale, and Cathy thought that she might well fit the description of a recent widow.

'Rosemary Holden? I'm so sorry to bother you. I'm Dr Moreland, from the Glainkirk Practice. I'm your registered GP, although I don't believe we've met.'

The other woman stepped back without speaking and turned, gesturing for Cathy to follow. With her back still to Cathy, she spoke.

'It's good of you to come. Not that I expected it. I suppose they inform you, do they? But I wasn't ... Thank you anyway. My mother's come to stay. She's just upstairs.'

Cathy closed the front door and followed her through.

'Your husband ...'

'Yes,' the woman said, leading Cathy into the front room. The room was bathed in light from the window and Cathy saw that along the mantlepiece was a line of condolence cards. She had been right after all.

'I'm so sorry.'

The woman gestured for Cathy to sit but didn't speak.

'It was David, wasn't it? He wasn't a patient of ours, but I had heard. How have you been doing? It was only at the weekend, I believe.'

She nodded.

Cathy sat in one of the armchairs. The room was immacu-late. She watched for a moment, considering the woman before her. She looked dreadful. Her hands were almost constantly moving and her face had a greyish hue.

'I've not been great, really. No. I was numb at the beginning. Maybe I am still. I can't seem to keep track of my thoughts, or the days even. That's normal, I assume?'

Cathy smiled. 'Anything goes,' she said. 'In my experience, grief can differ so greatly from person to person. Numbness is definitely up there and so is losing track of time.'

The other woman nodded. Her eyes flitted across Cathy's face and then up to the mantlepiece. In amongst the cards and flowers, was a collection of photographs.

'How are you sleeping?' Cathy asked and, to the woman's grimace, she nodded. 'I can prescribe something short term ...'

'I don't know. I don't want to sleep really. When I do, I have nightmares. It's almost better not to try.'

'I'll do a prescription,' Cathy said. 'It'll be at the pharmacy on the high street if you do decide you need it. Just a few days' worth.' She looked at Rosemary's dark eyes. 'Catnap when you can otherwise, and the same advice goes for eating. I realise that you're unlikely to be hungry, but graze on little bits of what you fancy. You said you had your mother staying?'

Rosemary nodded slightly.

'That's good. Better to have company now. You have friends also? I see from your notes that you only joined the practice a couple of years ago. Your husband ...'

'He didn't transfer,' the woman explained. 'We only moved from Forkieth. He didn't see the point.'

'I see. The police have been keeping you up to date with how things are progressing?'

'Yes. They've been quite kind. The funeral isn't going ahead yet. I think they're needing to do more tests. The gun wasn't right. They're speaking to the estate that ran the shoot. It wasn't David's gun. He borrowed one from the estate but then swapped it with one of the farmworkers.'

'Yes. I heard. I believe you know the Warrenders personally?'

The woman's face froze. Having been constantly moving, it was more exaggerated. Her features paled even further, if that was possible. Cathy shifted in her seat and began again. 'I'm sure it's been a difficult time for everyone ...'

To Cathy's astonishment, the woman snorted and let out what sounded like a laugh. She then covered her mouth. Her eyes became wild. Cathy knew she was on the verge of hysteria.

'It's alright,' she said. 'It's just the shock. Honestly. Can I get you something? A glass of water?'

The woman nodded but refused to allow her hands to drop from her mouth. Cathy hurried out of the room and found where the kitchen was, just off the hall. She ran the cold tap and having opened three cupboards, located the glasses. From the living room, she heard the woman sobbing. She glanced at the clock on the wall and saw that she would be cutting it fine to get back for the start of afternoon surgery. She quickly turned and then gasped as another woman stood in the doorway.

'Oh, sorry,' Cathy said. 'I was getting Mrs Holden a drink. I'm the doctor. I came past to check how she was doing. You must be her mother. She told me you were staying. Dr Moreland.' She reached out her hand to the other woman who took it in a cool grasp.

'I was just going really,' she admitted, now that the other woman had turned and retreated to the room in which Rosemary still sat.

Cathy handed Rosemary the water.

'I'll leave the prescription we discussed at the front desk of the surgery for you. Just in case you need it. Remember what I said. It will take a while to sink in, but if you feel it's overwhelming, please get in touch. I'll not bother you any longer. If I can do anything else at all, please let me know. My door's always open if you need to talk.'

Rosemary, whose face was now damp but expressionless, nodded.

The elderly woman saw her to the door.

'I doubt we'll need to bother you again, Doctor,' she said. 'Very nice of you to call, but it's family business now. If Rosemary needs to talk to anyone, it'll most likely be with me.'

Cathy smiled faintly and returned to her car with mixed feelings. As she drove back to the practice, she reflected on the encounter. Of course, she was glad finally to have met Mrs Holden. It helped to put a face to a name, and she had even managed to see a photograph of the dead man, on the mantlepiece. But if Cathy had hoped to uncover a potential killer in the young widow, it now seemed highly unlikely. Cathy thought of Rosemary's pale face and her fluttering hands. No, if ever there was a display of grief then that had been it. Cathy felt that she had gone awry somewhere. She must rethink the whole business.

35

Cathy sat in her room and stewed. Why had Rosemary Holden reacted so hysterically at the mention of the Warrenders? Was it simply a result of the general conversation about her husband's death, or was there something more? She considered all she knew about the case. David had wheedled his way onto the shoot at the last minute, from what Fiona had said. He had apparently little experience shooting and had only been able to take part under the supervision of the estate workers, including Gregory Warrender. Gregory, for whatever reason, had then offered the use of his own gun midway through the day. Up until then, Gregory had not shot. The rest of Glainkirk had jumped to the conclusion that he had doctored his gun and passed it to the other man, knowing full well that it might injure, if not kill. Mr Dewhurst had reasoned that the farmhand must have heard about David's company's plans. In attempting to buy over land and develop it for houses, they would disrupt Gregory's idyllic existence. He lived for his cattle and with the land sold off, it might all come to an end. But Cathy had no evidence to suggest that Gregory had known about David's scheme. David would hardly boast to Gregory about it, after all, when it was meant to be top secret. It wasn't even as if the pair were great friends.

Cathy wished she could find out what was said over the dinner table that night when the Warrenders and the Holdens met. Perhaps Fiona Warrender was her best bet if she wanted to know. Cathy sighed. It really wasn't the easiest. She had no right to be asking questions. Other than Mr Dewhurst's request, she had no reason to interfere.

No, it wasn't easy, and really her mind should be on other things. She thought again of the revalidation interview looming. She had still to pin down an exact date, and that day, she had received another reminder email from her assessor, suggesting that she and James come up with suggestions as her diary was filling up fast. Cathy looked out of her window. It was difficult to focus on anything just now. She found her mind returning to the fatal shooting.

The thing that bothered her the most was the mix-up with the guns. Why had they been swapped? It concerned her a good deal. But who could have known that the guns would be exchanged other than Gregory? It always came back to that. Well, Cathy thought to herself. If, for the sake of playing devil's advocate, she ruled Gregory out of the killing, how did that leave her? The only assumption was that David had not been the intended victim at all.

The phone on her desk rang.

'Sorry, Dr Moreland. I have a police inspector here at front reception. He wants to talk with you about the accident at the weekend. Are you able to see him just now?'

'Send him through, Michelle,' Cathy said and replacing the receiver, she sighed in resignation. What next? Had the police made any headway? They must surely have done a better job than her, that was for sure.

The police detective was a large, affable man. He was all

apologies for disturbing her and fumbled getting his notebook from his pocket and made a show of finding a pen. But Cathy watched and noted that his eyes were clear and his look attentive.

'Well then, Doctor,' he began. 'I suppose you know why I'm here? About the death up at the farm. I know the dead man wasn't a patient of yours, but our chief suspect is.'

'Oh?' Cathy asked, but of course, she knew who he must mean.

'A Mr Gregory Warrender.'

Cathy swallowed. 'Yes. He is a patient, as is his wife. I've seen them both recently.'

The police officer chuckled. 'Well, then. I'm already a step ahead there. I knew that, you see? Heard you'd even been out to do a house visit to the farm.'

Cathy blushed. 'They weren't actually at home when I called, as it happens.'

'I'll be straight with you, Doctor, if I may. I know that you're bound by confidentiality usually and so on, but I think you should know; Mr Warrender is this afternoon being questioned in the local police station. It is looking increasingly likely that he deliberately sabotaged his gun, forcing some metal object into the barrel, with the explicit purpose of injuring, if not killing David Holden. He has directed us to you. Not only as a character witness but because he apparently came in to have his gun licence renewed recently. I'd like to ask some questions regarding that, if you can answer?'

'If it's part of a criminal investigation, I have no option.'

The detective laughed. 'Right enough, but I like to be polite about things and not go crashing in, all the same. What can you tell me then? I assume that you do remember the consultation with Mr Warrender?'

'Oh yes,' Cathy said. 'I remember. I felt uncomfortable in some ways.'

The detective raised his bushy eyebrows.

'I'm not a great fan of guns,' she admitted. 'When he came in asking for the renewal, I couldn't really refuse. My senior partner is away this week. I did consider stalling, but he was adamant.'

'Threatening?'

'Oh no. I wouldn't go as far as that,' Cathy said. 'I did feel a bit manipulated though, but I had no reason not to sign really. He has no past medical history of psychiatric problems, no current thoughts of self-harm or low mood and no drug or alcohol abuse. I couldn't refuse on personal, ethical grounds without giving him an alternative doctor to seek the renewal from. To be honest, I didn't feel that strongly about the issue, I just dislike doing them.'

The detective smiled and nodded. 'No, I quite understand where you're coming from, and I agree.' He scribbled something in his notebook and Cathy waited. 'And to be sure,' he continued, glancing up. 'You had no reason to suspect that he was a danger to himself or others at all?'

Cathy swallowed. 'No proof whatsoever,' she said.

'Proof?' the detective asked, looking hard at her. 'But you had a suspicion?'

Cathy sighed. 'Not really even that. To be frank, I didn't warm to the man much. I've met his wife. She's a poor, frightened, little thing. Perhaps you've spoken with her already? I'll not go into why she came to see me, but I did see a bruise. It was on her arm.'

'Did you suspect domestic violence?'

Cathy wondered what she should answer. It was true, she had suspected just that and more. She recalled Fiona's wild accusation of Gregory poisoning her. 'Not really then, no, but ...'

'I know this is awkward for you Doctor, but I really must remind you that as part of a murder investigation, you are obliged to answer despite the oath of confidentiality. You've clearly changed your mind about the matter of Mr Warrender's risk to his wife. Can I ask why?'

Cathy sighed. 'His wife came in again after the shooting accident. She was generally anxious, which was understandable, I suppose. She made claims about being afraid, but not just of her husband, of the house she lived in. I didn't know what to think.'

'Does she believe her husband killed David Holden?'

'You'd have to ask her.'

'Your impression though?'

The room was completely silent. Outside, Cathy heard a car door slam. Time seemed to stand still. She looked again at the detective, knowing that her answer would only serve to further implicate Gregory Warrender, despite her doubts about him being involved in the crime.

'If pressed, then yes. I'd say that his wife does suspect her husband. That's not to say it's true though. I would say Fiona Warrender is an unreliable character. Since I've met her, she has been volatile.'

The detective smiled slightly and nodded. 'Can you give me any further information before I leave you in peace?'

Cathy shook her head. 'I think that's all I know. I had no reason to believe that Mr Warrender had been involved in the accident, and had no real reason to refuse to renew his gun licence. His wife may have her theories and she'd know him better than most, I suppose. I can't comment on that.'

The detective got up. 'Thanks for your time,' he said, moving to the door. 'Oh, just the one other thing ...'

Cathy looked up.

'The reason for the house call? You went out to visit the

Warrenders. That was directly after the weekend. Why was that, Doctor?'

Cathy felt sick. How was she to answer? She swallowed, but her mouth was dry. 'Just a courtesy visit, I suppose. I'd heard that there had been a fatal shooting at the weekend and it worried me.'

'I see,' the amiable policeman said. 'That seems in order then. You were checking to make sure Mr Warrender hadn't been somehow involved. Thank you, Doctor. You've been a great help.'

When he was gone, Cathy sat with her head in her hands. Oh God, what had she said?

36

Gregory shifted, trying to find a more comfortable position. The cold from the wall behind him seeped into his aching back. They had already asked him about the shoot. He had answered as best he could, but still, it didn't seem to satisfy them. He had thought that the policeman was on his side at the start. Asked him about the farm and so on, but when it came down to it, he was just like the rest of them. None of them believed him. Now, they were trying to keep him talking so that he might slip up in some way. He'd seen it done on the television. He'd explained himself time and again. There didn't seem any point in going over and over it. He felt sure that his words would be twisted to suit their purpose anyway. In the end, he'd stopped answering their questions. That was why he was sitting here now.

They'd offered him a solicitor at the start. Gregory had wondered about taking them up on this, but was that an admission of guilt? Would it only serve to compound their wild theories if he said yes? Gregory didn't know what to do for the best. He was trying to stay calm, but during the last hour of interviews, he had caught himself beginning to lose his temper. He supposed they had seen it too.

The hatch to the door opened.

'Mr Warrender?' a voice called.

Gregory looked up.

'Tea?'

Gregory shook his head and slouched back against the wall once more. Tea? Bloody joke it was. How could he sit and drink tea?

Although the hours in the police cell had depressed him, Gregory had tried to use the time well. At first, when they had closed the metal door, a sense of rising panic had almost consumed him. He had paced up and down angrily, but he was done with that now. He could hear echoes of people talking and moving about outside. They kept coming to check on him. When he wasn't being interviewed, they offered him refreshments and blankets too. The walls had initially seemed oppressive, but now, returning to the cell was a relief. He saw it as a quiet place to think. So much had happened since the shoot, that he had had little opportunity to do that.

A good deal of his thoughts centred around that fateful day. He knew that the deed had been done during the loss of Adam Foster's dog. It was the only time when everyone's attention was diverted. He had cursed himself a thousand times over for his stupidity in leaving the gun case either unlocked, or the keys sitting right next to it. What a gift it must have seemed to someone. The more he thought about it, the more certain Gregory became. Admittedly, over the years he had rubbed a few people up the wrong way, but this? To try to kill him? It seemed so extreme. Acceptance of this fact had not come easily, and Gregory had tried to make the story fit another way, but whatever way he looked at the thing, the gun backfiring could only have been meant for him. Who then? Who wanted him dead?

He cast his mind back to the events that day. Remembering the dash to the riverbank and then himself standing at the edge. Time and again, he had replayed the memory, visualising the faces that had flashed past as he ran from the field. He recalled also, standing on the river's edge and the hand on his back. A forceful shove. It had definitely been deliberate. Someone had wanted him to fall into the fast-flowing water. They had wanted to endanger him, perhaps hoping that he too might die along with Adam's dog. That same person had meddled with his gun. Having failed to drown him, it had been the next best thing.

Gregory shook his head. He'd not seen the face of the man in the bushes, it was true, but he had noticed something much later.

Gregory's head lolled back against the cold stone of the wall. He looked at the blank ceiling and smiled. Then, despite the seriousness of his predicament, he snorted. Rocking forward, his body suddenly convulsed with heaves of noiseless laughter, until the tears rolled down, stinging his cheeks. Oh God, but if it was so, it only meant one thing. He was as well being arrested and charged because he had lost everything anyway.

37

Cathy knew the caller before they spoke. She heard the intake of breath. 'Mrs Warrender?'

'Yes. Yes, it's me. I'm sorry. Oh God, it's always me, bothering people. I didn't know who else to call. My sister's not talking to me. Even she thinks he did it. So does my mum. The police came. They've taken him away. Locked him in a cell. Everyone saw. The farmworkers, Adam Foster, even old Mr Dewhurst. They were all standing watching. It was awful. I didn't know what to do. It's such a mess. I should have been back at work today, but ... Oh God! I don't even know what I'm saying. My head, you see? I'm so confused and when I try to think; the pain!'

'Calm down, Fiona,' Cathy said, and immediately realised how stupid a request this was. The girl's words had been slurred. If she hadn't been drinking, she was quite hysterical. 'I've just had a police officer in here seeing me. He seemed quite sensible. He's trying to find out the facts. Gregory isn't under arrest. They are simply interviewing him.'

Cathy could hear the woman sniffing and there was a muffled sound at the other end of the line. 'I know all that, but they'll find out, you see? They're clever, the police. What if he is guilty? What if he killed David? They'll know. Everyone already knows. Oh, God! Poor Rosemary won't even see me now. She can't stand the sight of me! I don't know what to do. I've made the most terrible mistake. Oh God, what have I done?'

Cathy sat up straight in her chair. 'Fiona? Now listen. What have you done?'

There was more sobbing. 'Oh God. How was I to know it would turn out like this? No-one could know, could they?'

Cathy spoke firmly. 'Fiona, I want you to listen to me now. Where are you?'

'Here, I'm here. I'm always here. There are mice, there are rats. Sometimes I feel like they're in the walls laughing me!'

'Stay where you are. I'll be with you in fifteen minutes.'

She hung up the phone and marched from her room.

'Michelle,' she said as she passed the front desk. 'Emergency call out to Glainkirk Farm. Get Linda to see any others that come in and apologise for me please.'

The lead receptionist looked up startled. 'Alright, Dr Moreland. I hope it's nothing serious.'

Cathy didn't reply, but hurried to her car, her doctors' bag in hand. She had a dreadful feeling that Fiona Warrender might either have taken something she shouldn't or now be at high risk of doing so.

It seemed to take an eternity to get there. The roads were narrow and winding and at one point, Cathy found herself stuck behind a tractor. The driver realised that she was in a hurry though, and signalled, then pulling into a field entrance and allowing her to pass. Cathy remembered the first time she had driven this route, only a week or so ago when she had crashed into a ditch and met Gregory Warrender. So much had happened since.

The house was in darkness when she arrived. Feeling rising

panic, she parked her car and grabbing her bag from the back seat, jogged across the lane to the house.

'Mrs Warrender?' she called as she knocked for the second time. 'Please come to the door. It's the doctor. I need to speak to you.' She tried the handle but it wouldn't budge.

Cathy moved around the side of the cottage, looking in the windows as she did so. She paused at the kitchen window and jumped, seeing Fiona sitting with her head on the kitchen table. Cathy banged on the window.

'Fiona! Open the door now!'

The girl didn't raise her head. Cathy looked wildly about her and then ran around the house to the back door. She tried the handle, but it wouldn't give either. Cathy hammered on the door and shouted. Running back around the house, she saw a car drawing up and prayed they might help.

'I need to get inside,' she said breathlessly to the driver. His car was in the middle of the road, but he opened the door and got out. 'What is it? What's happened?'

'I need to get in. I was about to smash a window. I think she's taken something.'

'Oh shit!' The man strode up the path in front of Cathy. 'Fiona open this door!' he shouted. He turned back to Cathy. 'I have spare keys in the office. It'd take five minutes.'

Cathy looked doubtful.

'I'll smash it in then,' he said and put his shoulder to the door.

After the third attempt, the wood made a dreadful splintering sound. It took two more runs at it, and then he was in. Cathy pushed past and found the door to the kitchen. The girl was slumped and quite insensible. There was a bottle of port on the table. The smell of alcohol was overwhelming.

'Fiona! Wake up! I need you to wake up!'

Cathy lifted a strand of limp hair from the girl's face. Her eyelids were almost blue and closed tight shut, her cheeks a deep red. Her face had a look of passivity. Cathy gently felt for a carotid pulse. 'She's still with us. Can you call for an ambulance? I don't know if she's taken anything on top of the drink.'

While he did this, Cathy continued to try to get the girl to wake. She crossed the room and opened the back door and the windows. The cold air was startling and this at least seemed to rouse Fiona. The young woman groaned.

'Good,' Cathy said, feeling both relief and anger.

Fiona shifted and her eyes fluttered.

'Fiona. I need you to tell me if you've swallowed anything. Fiona, open your eyes for me now.'

The girl's forehead creased into a frown and she moaned again. Then, with some effort, she licked her lips. 'Sorry,' she slurred. 'I'm an idiot.'

The man returned to the room. Cathy had heard him giving directions to the ambulance telephone operator.

'Should be here soon. Is she OK?'

'I don't know. She's conscious at least. I'll have a quick scout around to see if I can find any empty pill packets.'

'Right. I'll help look upstairs,' he said. 'I'm Adam, by the way, the estate manager. What a day it's been for us.'

Cathy grimaced and they began their search, with Cathy reluctant to leave the girl's sight in case she deteriorated. In the kitchen anyway, she found nothing of interest. She even tentatively looked into the bin, but no foil packet or bottle was evident.

'Anything?' she asked, as Adam came back downstairs. He shook his head.

'I'm so sorry,' Fiona slurred once more from her position at the table. She raised her head and squinted. 'What a bloody mess.'

'She's right about that,' Adam said. 'First Gregory and now this.'

They heard the scream of sirens as the ambulance approached. The estate manager went out and waved, showing the crew where to pull in and park up behind his car.

'I'd better move,' he said, coming in once more to Cathy. 'Looks like they want to get the ambulance closer to the door. Are you alright? I'll be at the estate office all afternoon if you need me. I'll send someone out to see to the door later.'

Cathy thanked him and then, as the paramedics came in, she focused her attention on handing over to them, giving them as much detail as she possibly could. When Fiona was strapped into a chair, her knees covered by blankets, Cathy knelt beside her.

'Fiona? Look at me. We'll sort this out, OK? Everything will work out. Now, you concentrate on getting better and help the doctors in A and E by telling them what you took, alright? I'll call the hospital later and see how you're doing.'

Cathy straightened up and thanked the paramedics. She stood in the kitchen alone, watching as the young woman, so pale and fragile, was wheeled up the ramp into the back of the ambulance. Fiona had been right in what she had said. It was indeed a mess. Cathy felt more determined than ever now to get to the bottom of things. She knew that half of Glainkirk, apparently along with his wife, believed Gregory Warrender guilty of murder. She had disliked him personally also, but that didn't diminish the fact that the gun that had been tampered with had been his. If Gregory hadn't been the killer, it only meant one thing: he had been the real target. If that was so, the killer had, through Gregory's insistence in handing his gun to David, accidentally killed the wrong man. Cathy frowned. Although it was awful that Gregory was in police custody, it did mean that for now at least, he was safe. But if the farm labourer was released, did it put him in danger again, and what of his wife, who had repeatedly apologised in her drunken stupor, and told Cathy that she had made a dreadful mistake?

She pulled what was left of the Warrenders' front door closed and stood for a moment, watching the ambulance wend its way along the narrow lanes. A difficult journey at the best of times, but more so in a hurry. Cathy began to walk down the garden path to her car. She moved her doctors' bag to the other hand as she came to the gate. Was she missing an opportunity?

Slowly, Cathy retraced her steps, glancing back as she did so. No-one was about and what she was doing was legitimate. Mr Dewhurst had specifically asked her to look into the fatal shooting for him. It was, at the end of the day, his house. The Warrenders just rented it. Cathy felt her heart rate quicken as she closed the door behind her. Where first? Upstairs? It was cold, as they had thrown all the windows open earlier. Cathy shivered. She needed to hurry. But she didn't know quite what she was looking for. Evidence to either implicate or exonerate Gregory or his wife. But what form that might take, she wasn't sure.

She climbed the stairs, glancing from side to side as she did so. Coming to the landing, she was faced with three closed doors. She touched each, knowing that they must all be empty, but afraid all the same, of what she might find. Ridiculous. Gregory was at the police station and Fiona, on the way to the hospital. She had nothing to fear. Cathy pushed the first door. It was the main bedroom. The duvet lay messily across the double mattress and the bedside tables were in disarray. Fiona certainly wasn't house-proud, that was for sure. The estate manager must have looked in here already when he was searching for any tablets that Fiona might have swallowed. Cathy looked around the room, unsure where to begin.

The chest of drawers was covered in an assortment of makeup accessories, with compacts and lipsticks lying haphazardly by a mirror. Fiona, it was true, had always been well dressed and had taken pride in her appearance. The top drawer of the chest revealed nothing of any great surprise. Cathy felt disgusted at herself as she turned over underwear. She hastily replaced everything she had moved and quickly searched the other drawers. Nothing. The thought of going through the bedside cabinets didn't appeal, but for the sake of thoroughness, she did open the doors to each. Other than a packet of condoms and a tatty-looking romance novel, she found nothing. She had hoped to find a diary, but then who even had one these days? If she thought Fiona was going to pen her deepest feelings for a lover, and then leave the book for Gregory to find, she was being very naive indeed. Cathy shook her head in disappointment.

She moved on from the main bedroom and tried the room adjacent. A spare bedroom, but it looked as if it had been slept in recently. Perhaps the Warrenders had fallen out and were using separate rooms. Cathy thought of the packet of condoms next door and wondered when they were last utilized, perhaps not for a while given the current state of play. She gave the room she was in the same attention as the last. At the dressing table, Cathy pulled out a drawer and found a flat, wooden box, perhaps the size of one of her large medical textbooks. She opened it. Old coins and a few bits of bronze-looking metal. Was one of the Warrenders a collector? She closed the lid and moved on. There was nothing in the bedside cabinet other than a box of tissues. How frustrating.

Cathy moved to the final room on the first floor, which she had rightly assumed was the bathroom. It was a small room with a shower and no bath. Again, Cathy supposed that the estate manager must have looked in here too. There was a multitude of hair products, but no sign of a pill bottle. Cathy now doubted if Fiona had swallowed anything other than alcohol. Only time would tell. She might telephone the hospital later and find out.

For completeness, Cathy checked the small pedal-bin in the corner, a couple of cardboard toilet roll tubes but no pill bottle. Cathy was about to let the lid fall when she spotted a printed piece of paper. It had slid along the edge of the plastic bag that the Warrenders had used as a bin liner. Presumably, they lifted this entirely when changing the bin. She had a similar setup herself. She stooped and recovered the discarded sheet of paper. It was folded over and Cathy immediately recognised it as a patient information leaflet, the kind always included in boxes of medicine detailing the potential side-effects and recommended dosage of a drug. She read the treatment name and nodded. So, her suspicions had been correct. Fiona had been edgy when she asked about her menstrual cycle and it had been for a reason. In her hand, Cathy held the leaflet for Levonorgestrel, the morning after pill. Not prescribed by her, but the emergency contraceptive was quite easy to acquire directly from a pharmacist now without it ever being recorded in a patient's medical records. It seemed highly suggestive, given that Fiona had failed to divulge this to her when she might easily have done so. Well, Cathy thought, descending the stairs, it wasn't such a great surprise anyway. She had thought that Fiona was playing a dangerous game, and she already knew with whom. The gamekeeper Kenneth was the only person it could be unless Fiona had someone else on the go at her work.

Cathy made a quick tour of the downstairs of the house. She saw that under the kitchen sink was a container marked with hazard stickers. Rat poison, by the looks of it. Nasty stuff and silly to keep it in the kitchen. She found little else of interest, but she did find where Gregory had kept his gun, in a brown, leather case, now empty of course, under the stairs along with an old metal-detector and a whole host of nasty-looking wellington boots. It all seemed secure enough though and Cathy, already twitchy about the time she was taking, closed the door to the cupboard and made her way out of the house.

As she drove back to the practice, she thought about her search. Did her discovery confirm that Fiona was having an affair with Kenneth? Perhaps not, but if she and Gregory were indeed sleeping in separate beds, it did pose the question as to why the girl needed the pill. If Kenneth was her lover, it put both parties in the frame she supposed. If ever there was a likely motive for killing Gregory, adultery must surely be high up there. Had Fiona so desperately hated her brute of a husband? Had she been sick of his rough treatment and desperate for an escape, to perhaps make a new life for herself with the gamekeeper? Was it possible that this had driven her to take drastic action? And what of Kenneth himself? Had the man struggled to watch his lover's confidence diminish? Had he seen the bruises on the young woman's arms and in fury, tampered with Gregory's gun, knowing that the man would shoot it that fateful day? He had been there at the shoot, after all. The gamekeeper, standing coldly on the sidelines. Had he watched Gregory as he collected his gun that afternoon? What horror must he have felt on seeing the wrong man take it, and then the inevitable? Cathy felt sick even thinking about it.

Thankfully, it seemed that nothing urgent had come in while she had been away rummaging around the Warrenders' house. Just as well. It wouldn't look good right before her revalidation to have a significant event on her hands. It was after half-past six when she finished her paperwork for the day following an afternoon consulting. Wearily, she dialled for an outside line and waited for the operator to put her through.

'Well darling,' Suzalinna said. 'I didn't expect to hear your lovely voice today. When they said a GP was on the line asking for me, my heart sank, to be honest. Another daft referral. When they insist on speaking to the consultant rather than the registrar, it never bodes well, does it? Anyway, what can I do for you? I assume you want something.'

Cathy laughed. 'Sorry to bother you at work. I'm wondering if you had an update on a query overdose I sent in? It was the girl I was speaking to you about before, Fiona Warrender?'

'Not one I've seen. I've been busy in resus all afternoon with a brittle asthmatic, but hang on a sec.' Cathy heard her friend calling across the room. There was a mumbling of voices and the receiver crackled. Cathy imagined her friend dressed in surgical scrubs, holding her hand over the phone.

'Hi, Cathy? Yes, it's one Frances saw. She's waiting on paracetamol levels coming back. Your girl denies taking anything though. Spewed her guts up and made a fine mess of bay four apparently. Just booze, by the looks of it, unless you know something we don't?'

'Not really. I checked the house properly after the ambulance left. I found rat poison under the sink. Might be worthwhile doing a clotting screen and LFTs, I suppose, but you've probably done that already.'

'Right you are,' Suzalinna said. 'She's heading up to the short-stay ward in a bit. Frances said there was no-one at home or she might have discharged her this evening if the bloods were normal.'

'Suz, do me a favour, will you?'

'Sure.'

'Just give Frances a heads up. I found the morning after pill in her bin. Might be worthwhile double-checking she's definitely not pregnant.'

'OK. Anything else? I hope you're not too involved in all of this, Cathy? This isn't related in some way to your little investigation into the fatal shooting, is it? We agreed that you were leaving it to the police ...'

Cathy laughed. 'Bye Suz, I have to get on.'

Cathy hung up to Suzalinna's ill-tempered retort.

She needed to go home and get something to eat. All the business with Fiona had meant that she had missed lunch. Certainly, she would have to look into the thing further. She knew where she must concentrate her efforts. It seemed incredible that she had not started there. If she was to find out exactly what happened on the day of the shoot, she needed to speak to the right people. Gregory and Fiona were of no use to her currently but, now she had met the man, she felt that the best way forward was with Adam, the estate manager. If anyone had watched the events unfolding without bias, it must surely be him.

Adam cleared his throat. 'And you say Mr Dewhurst ...?'
'Feel free to check first,' Cathy said. 'He specifically asked that I make a few informal inquiries. I know it seems odd, really, I do. I think we all want this dreadful business concluded as fast as possible though, no matter how it's gone about. I've heard from the hospital about Fiona Warrender. She should be home later today. Thank you for your help yesterday, by the way. I might have broken a window instead of forcing the door if I'd been on my own. If I had done that, I could well have ended up in accident and emergency myself needing stitches.'

Adam seemed to relax. 'No, that's alright. I went back and patch up the door later on. It'll need to be replaced anyway. Someone's coming out to look at it. That house is a mess. I need to speak to Mr Dewhurst, not that he'll be pleased.'

'Money issues?' Cathy probed.

Adam shot her a look. 'Mr Dewhurst's alright. It's always tricky when there's so much in the way of land and properties on it.'

'He has how many acres?'

'Near enough a hundred.'

'I had no idea. It must be quite something managing it all. Have you always worked here?'

'Just the last five years. I did some estate work up one of the glens. Mainly property management. Dealing with the rented places and arranging for large shooting parties to be accommodated. It was fine enough, but I fancied a change.'

'Oh, so the shooting isn't a new thing for you?'

Adam shook his head. 'No, not at all. On the other estate, it was deer.'

Cathy sniffed.

'Not everyone's cup of tea,' the estate manager said as if understanding. 'A way of life really, especially if you've been brought up with it.'

'I suppose so. Well, certainly a way of life for Gregory Warrender.'

'Greg was a good enough shot. Didn't have the heart for it though. I couldn't blame him, to be fair. Sometimes it's tiresome teaching these folks coming to the estate. Some of them are good. Many of them aren't. The worst ones have done a bit of shooting in the past and think they know it all. They're the ones to keep an eye on.'

'Not like the man who died though. I hear he was a complete novice.'

Adam nodded. 'He was fine. Nervous and didn't have the patience to really get to grips with it. If he'd come back and had a few more lessons, he'd have settled maybe. Not a natural though.'

'You were supervising him a good deal that day?'

'I was. I always look after the novices.'

'You carry your own gun too?'

'No. I'm too focused on other things. Gregory and some of the others brought theirs that day. I check their paperwork obviously before we start. Greg's was all in order that morning. As far as I knew, he didn't shoot at all. Kept his gun in the boot of the jeep. That was all as it should have been too. I don't like guns lying about and if they're not in use, they have to be kept in the cars in their cases.'

'Sounds sensible enough,' Cathy said. 'So, at lunchtime, all the guns would be back in the cars?'

'That's correct.'

'And the man who died? His gun would have been in Gregory's car beside his own?'

'Oh no. He had been shooting with me, you see? His gun was in my boot.'

'But the people Gregory had overseen that morning?'

'Yes, their guns were in beside his, I assume. We have our own estate cases. All the guns would have been in those. I'll show you one if you like?' He got up and went to the office door. Cathy waited. When he returned, he was holding a long, rectangular box. He placed it on the table. 'We keep these in the gun cabinets next door and those are locked too. Extra safety precaution.'

Cathy nodded. 'So, your cases all have the estate stamp embossed on them?' she asked, running her fingers across the black, leather case and the family crest. '*Invicta veritate*,' Cathy read aloud. 'I was rubbish at Latin,' she laughed.

'By invincible truth,' Adam translated.

Cathy imagined old Mr Dewhurst's ancestors charging into battle with this war cry, and shivered. 'So, all the gun cases look alike?' she asked. 'How did you keep track of who was using each gun?'

Adam turned the case around and Cathy saw a serial number.

'Guns and cases match up. Each person was assigned a number at the beginning of the day and they were told not to swap.'

Cathy grimaced. 'But Greg and David did.'

Adam shook his head. 'It was against protocol. I've no idea why he swapped. We've spoken to him about it but it's to him to explain that to the police now.'

Cathy nodded. At least she had gleaned one thing so far from what Adam had said. She had already seen Gregory's gun case in the cupboard below his stairs. It looked quite different from these estate cases, so any chance of mistaken identity and another gun being the target of vandalism now seemed wholly unlikely.

'So, Gregory would have overseen his group all morning?'

'We shot in a different area in the morning and moved to the second drive before lunch. The idea was that we could start up straight after without messing around.'

'I see.'

'Greg's group had done better than we anticipated. One of them was talking about shooting across the river so I think he was going to allow that. Potter's Field is a bit of a favourite with our shooters. If they've been with us before, they'll often ask to go there again. I was still overseeing another group and then Kenny, our gamekeeper, came at lunch and offered to help too.'

'And other people joined you for lunch?'

'I saw Gregory's wife came along, and David's too, I believe. They were off in a group chatting. The beaters sometimes have their families join them also. It's a long day otherwise.'

Cathy grimaced. Of course, she had completely forgotten that there would be people driving the birds out of the undergrowth as well as the estate staff manning the shoot.

'Are the beaters all estate employees?' she asked.

'No, some are from the town. It's a quick buck. If they're

manual workers, at this time of the year, money's hard to come by. Some of them come back year after year. A few of the people who shoot tip them if they do a nice job.'

Cathy nodded. 'I see. That all makes sense. So, can you tell me a bit about the afternoon shoot? Mr Dewhurst has filled me in a little, but you were running it, and probably in a better position than most to see what happened.'

But Adam shook his head. 'I can tell you about the morning, but I wasn't there when the accident happened. Neither was Mr Dewhurst.'

'Oh?' Cathy asked, now puzzled.

'Seems insignificant now, after a man lost his life, but my dog. She was one of my prize bitches. Bred three litters from her. All went to shooting homes.'

Cathy waited.

'My fault really,' Adam admitted, shrugging his shoulders. 'Shouldn't have let them out of the jeep over lunch, but they're usually fine. Got buzzed up with everyone laughing and carrying on, I suppose. Gregory's wife was one of the loudest, I seem to recall. I didn't know it had happened until someone shouted. Fell into the river at the bottom of the field,' he explained. 'It runs pretty fast when it's high and the night before it had rained. Must have been chasing a bird or what have you. Fell in and couldn't get back out. I sprinted over, but she was already floundering. I couldn't get down the side.' The estate manager looked distraught recounting the story. 'In the end, it was Gregory who went in to try and get her. Ran down the side of the field and tried to catch her. I was way behind, but I think some of the others were helping him. When the old girl was lost, I'm afraid I fairly went to pieces. Mr Dewhurst took me up to the big house and gave me a whisky. We came back after half an hour, but only arrived to see the man lying there dead.'

Cathy nodded. If ever there was a perfect opportunity to meddle with Gregory's gun as it lay unattended in the back of his car, then the confusion surrounding the drowned dog at lunchtime was surely it.

'Adam, can you try to remember for me? When your dog fell in, were you at the back of the group then? I assume everyone gathered by the river to see if they could help?'

Adam screwed up his face in concentration, 'Who was in front of me?' he asked himself. 'Well, Mr Dewhurst was following me, I do know that. He took longer to walk. The ground's uneven and he had his stick. I know that David was there, pretty much all of the beaters too.'

'What about Gregory's wife?' Cathy asked.

Adam grimaced. 'You know, I can't say for sure. She was about. I did hear her calling. She's got an annoying sort of a tone to her voice,' he laughed, and then his face straightened. 'She was calling for Gregory to do something at the start, but then I think she was close by. I heard her sort of whispering.'

Cathy held her breath.

'Kind of hissing at him, she was. 'Do it, do it now,' she was saying. I think we were all saying much the same. Gregory was standing out in the river and not moving. He could have got to the dog if he'd just moved faster. Time was a bit frozen for me. Think it was the shock of the whole thing. Loved that dog, I did. I've felt wretched about it since.'

Cathy thanked the estate manager. She had learned a good deal from him, not least what Fiona had been overheard saying. Admittedly, Adam had assumed she was urging Gregory to hurry up. Well, anyone at the time might have assumed that's was what she had meant, but what if she had been speaking to someone else? What if she had been instructing someone? Telling them to hurry up while the focus of the group was on something else? Cathy could only guess to whom she might have been talking. Undoubtedly the next person she must speak with, was Kenneth, the gamekeeper. What had been so vital for him to 'do now?'

40

A s Cathy was driving out of the estate, she wondered if Gregory, or indeed his wife, might now be home. Instead of continuing, she swung the car right at the junction and drove up the track to the Warrenders' house. It would be foolish to return to Glainkirk only to hear that Fiona was out of hospital and needing a follow-up home visit.

She parked outside the house and saw that a light was on. Cathy checked her mobile. When she had left the practice that morning, she had told Michelle to let her know of any urgent calls. Well, Michelle hadn't left any messages, so she assumed she was fine until eleven when her first patients were booked in.

Cathy crossed the track and pushed open the gate to the cottage. As she neared, she saw the temporary repairs Adam had made to the front door and grimaced. A horrible reminder of what had happened only the day before. The door was opened, but not by either of the Warrenders.

'Back again?' he asked.

Cathy blushed. 'I assume Fiona's home? May I come in, I'm her doctor.'

He stepped back and gestured for her to come into the hall.

'So that's who you are,' he said. 'Well, Doctor, your patient is through here, in the living room. Fi, you've got an unexpected visitor.'

Cathy followed Kenneth through the hallway, and when he opened the door to the room and ushered her inside, she realised that she had done a rather foolish thing. She had allowed him, a man currently high on her list of suspects for the attempted murder of Gregory, and accidental killing of David, to stand between her and the only exit from the cottage. Cathy clenched her jaw and decided that she must go along with things for now, and hopefully find a way to position herself better during the conversation. Part of her still couldn't believe that either he or Fiona was a killer though but it didn't do any harm being cautious.

Fiona was lying on the sofa with a tartan rug pulled up over her legs. The television was blaring in the corner. Cathy doubted that the girl was even watching it. She looked wan and brittle, perhaps more so than yesterday when Cathy had watched her wheeled into the ambulance.

'Fiona?' she said and the girl turned and looked confused as if she hadn't realised that anyone was there.

'Oh, it's you,' she said and turned back to the television screen.

'Fiona, I was passing the cottage and I wanted to see how you were. Can we turn the sound down?'

Kenneth strode across the room and flicked the switch by the plug. 'There,' he said. 'I'll be in the kitchen if you need me, Fiona.'

Cathy wondered at the man's audacity, behaving in such a way, especially in another man's house. All the same, she was glad that she and Fiona were alone, although she wondered how closely her lover might be listening at the door.

'I wanted to follow up after what happened yesterday,' Cathy began. 'I've not had the discharge sheet from the hospital yet. How are you feeling about things now?'

Fiona didn't look at her and remained silent.

Cathy sighed and sat down on the edge of one of the chairs. 'Fiona, please speak. I'm only trying to help. You were very distressed when we last spoke. Have you had thoughts of harming yourself in the past? I had wondered if you'd swallowed something yesterday ...'

The girl's hands fidgeted in her lap.

'Listen, I know things have been stressful for you. I don't doubt that yesterday, it came to a head when Gregory was taken in for questioning. You've been frightened for a long time, I believe.'

The hands froze.

'I'm right, aren't I? Fiona, really, I can't help if you won't talk. I'm glad you have some support. I take it you and he are ...'

The girl turned. 'Oh, you would think that.' Her eyes narrowed and Cathy was horrified to see how savagely she spoke.

'I – Look, it doesn't matter. I wanted to make sure you were safe. If you need to talk about anything, we have people who can help. I don't know what the hospital has recommended but if you do need to be referred on, I'll see to it.' Cathy sighed, seeing Fiona's face return to passivity. 'Have you heard from Gregory?'

She thought there was a flash of emotion in the girl's eyes, but she didn't answer.

'Look, I'll leave you if you're sure that's what you want?'

Again, there was no response.

Cathy rose and went to the door. 'I'm here for you if you need anything. If you'd rather not deal with me, there are other doctors at the surgery.'

Cathy felt quite sick, thinking of leaving the girl in such an odd state.

In the hallway, she was met by Kenneth.

'I assume she wasn't feeling too communicative?'

'Are you going to be keeping an eye on her today?' Cathy asked.

'I've work to do, but I'll be popping back and forward.'

Cathy nodded. 'That's fine. I assume she's not said anything to you about ...' but she trailed off, not knowing how to ask.

'About Gregory?'

'Well, any of it, I suppose. I think she's in a very vulnerable state at the moment. I am genuinely concerned.'

The gamekeeper's face softened. Surely he and Fiona couldn't have plotted to kill her husband. They might well be having an affair behind Gregory's back, but to try to murder him, and in cold blood? It seemed too far-fetched.

'Listen, before I go, you were there when the man was fatally wounded,' Cathy said. 'Why did he and Gregory swap guns? I just can't understand it.'

'God knows,' he replied and lifted the fringe of curls from his forehead in a sweeping gesture. 'I was surprised Gregory was even on speaking terms with the man. Made himself as obnoxious to everyone else as he could.'

Cathy was puzzled. She had heard that Gregory had been unpleasant to Fiona, but not anyone else.

'Who had he fallen out with?' she asked.

'Well, me, for a start. Can't blame him much for that I suppose, but everyone around was sick of his ill-temper. At lunchtime, he made himself out to be a right fool. Fiona was humiliated. Her friend tried to smooth things over.'

'Oh?' Cathy asked. 'Who was that?'

'The woman. The one whose husband died. Rosemary. She was there over lunch. Think it was as much to give Fi moral support as to come and see her own husband. I got the feeling she knew, if you see what I mean? She was trying to help. I suppose Fiona must have confided in her about Gregory. She made a joke out of his ridiculous sulking. Well, we all did to make it less awkward, but you could tell Fiona was embarrassed.'

'And during lunch, Fiona was where?'

'Oh, well with us, she was in a big group.' Kenneth took a step towards Cathy. 'Listen, I hope you're not implying that Fiona's a suspect. I can guarantee she wasn't alone for a second during that shoot.'

'I'd better get back to the surgery,' Cathy said and made for the door.

But Kenneth stepped forward, barring her exit.

Cathy's heart quickened and she suddenly felt faint.

'Doctor. I'm worried about Fiona,' he said earnestly. They were only inches apart in the already cramped hall. An overwhelming sense of unease settled over Cathy, but the gamekeeper was talking again. 'If you meant what you said about genuinely wanting to help,' he said and stepped in even closer. His voice was now a whisper. 'She was alright on the way back from the hospital. I collected her; you see? Brightest I've seen her in a while. Tired, as you might expect, but her face looked somehow, less troubled. This morning though. I've not been with her the whole time, had to go in and out to the pheasants, but ... Well, you saw her just now. She seems to have gone back a step. She's so jumpy and sometimes I wonder if she can even hear what I'm saying.'

'I can't do much unless she–'

'I know all that,' he said angrily and slapped the wall with the palm of his hand. 'I don't want Gregory to come back home and for things to get worse. Do you know what I mean, Doctor, or are we on a completely different wavelength?'

Cathy didn't know what he meant, but in the cramped hallway, she was becoming increasingly desperate to get outside.

'I really must go,' she said again. 'Please let me pass.'

Kenneth didn't move.

Cathy's heart was now pounding in her ears. In a moment of desperation, she rushed at the man and threw herself on the door, scrabbling at the handle.

It opened and she almost fell onto the step outside.

'Doctor?' he called, but Cathy was stumbling down the path, her head throbbing. Perhaps Fiona had been right after all. The house was cursed, or maybe it was Kenneth. Cathy didn't know what it was, but she knew she had to get away.

41

R osemary sat by the window. A car had pulled up outside. It was one she had seen before. She got up and walked to the door, opening it mechanically.

'You came back?' she asked and stepped aside.

'May I come in?' Dr Moreland asked, which seemed unnecessary as Rosemary had already turned and begun walking towards the living room.

'My mother's gone out,' she said. 'I don't think either of us could stand one another any longer. I suppose families are like that, even at times of stress. She came to comfort me, but she's done little of that. We've fallen comfortably back into our roles, despite me being an adult and now widowed.'

Rosemary sat down and clasped her hands together. So many people had come to the house, she hardly knew which one was which and what she had said to them all. Why she was talking so superficially with complete strangers was beyond her.

The doctor crossed to the mantlepiece and glanced at one of David's photos. Rosemary wondered if she was going to pick up a card she had been sent by her employers, but she turned instead.

'I've been concerned about you.'

Rosemary nodded and smiled. 'Everyone's been so kind. I didn't take any of your tablets. Perhaps I should have done. Sleeping's been difficult. Everything's been difficult. I suppose you're used to this. Used to dealing with people when they're like this. I wonder how long it will go on; feeling this way.'

She glanced up and the doctor was smiling sadly. 'I've just been to the Warrenders' house,' she said.

Rosemary's stomach lurched. She didn't want to hear about the Warrenders. If she never heard the name again, she would be only too happy.

'Fiona Warrender has been unwell herself,' the doctor was saying.

Rosemary frowned. She didn't want to listen to it but the other woman kept talking. Who did she think she was, coming back to her house? She hadn't asked her to come. She'd never even consulted her before all this.

'I don't know if you've heard, but Fiona's husband, Mr Warrender, has been taken in for questioning by the police?'

Rosemary's hands shook and she clasped them tighter. When would this end?

'You were friends, before all of this?'

'With her, yes,' Rosemary conceded.

'I understand that Gregory wasn't universally liked?'

Rosemary grimaced at the understatement. 'I've no idea how she put up with him. I'm glad he's been arrested. I hope they find out the truth about what he did, the manipulative bastard.'

The doctor crossed the room and sat beside her. Rosemary was aware of her heart beating rapidly.

'Can I ask a little about that day?'

'The shoot? I don't mind talking,' Rosemary said defiantly. In truth, she wanted to be alone and never to speak of it again.

'You went for lunch, I believe? I've spoken with one of the estate staff. He told me that a group of you were standing chatting over the break between shoots.'

Rosemary nodded, In her mind, she saw David laughing. He threw his head back and bared his teeth when he laughed. He always had beautiful teeth. The woman was waiting for an answer.

'Yes, that's right,' she stammered. 'We were all together. Fiona and I brought a picnic. I'd made a quiche.'

A wave of nausea crashed over her at the thought of the food.

'There was an accident with a dog?'

Rosemary nodded. 'Yes. It drowned. Everyone was quite upset.'

'None more so than the dog's owner.'

'Adam. Yes, he seemed nice enough.'

'Not according to Gregory, it seems.'

'Gregory had a grievance with everyone. He had an inferiority complex of sorts. But you're wrong in what you say. On the previous evening, Fiona told me that it had all changed. There was a miraculous transformation between them, just days before the shoot. Gregory got a promotion, it seems. Boasted that he'd be bringing home more money every month.'

'I wonder why.'

'I don't know,' Rosemary said, considering it for the first time. 'Adam had been round to the house apparently, so Fiona said. Goodness knows how the pair of them found any common ground after years of apparently hating one another. Fiona used to tell me all about it.' Rosemary sighed. The train commute seemed a lifetime ago. 'Adam was seemingly keen at dishing out demands, but Gregory wasn't too good at taking orders.'

'But they called a truce?'

Rosemary looked out of the window. She was now thinking of the train journey to work. She recalled her and Fiona Warrender's giggled conversations. And then she again remembered the old woman who had sat beside her on the day Fiona had missed the train. That had been the beginning of things. That had changed everything, she thought.

42

Cathy was horrified to discover that Michelle had in fact tried to phone her twice while she had been visiting Rosemary Holden. Apparently, Mr Duncan, the elderly gentleman whom Cathy had inadvertently offended when she last visited, had phoned requesting an urgent house call.

By the time Cathy got to the sheltered housing complex, there was already an ambulance outside.

'What happened?' she asked the paramedic as they closed the doors.

'Chest pains. Doesn't sound cardiac at all, but you never can tell. ECG wasn't good enough quality really. We'll take him in for a check over. House is in a bit of a state. Doubt he'll get home without a bit more backup.'

Cathy felt sick as she watched the ambulance turn. Oh, God. Had she failed Mr Duncan so dreadfully as this? But she hadn't known about the state of the house or the chest discomfort. He should have called her sooner and she might have helped him more. What a mess she had made of things and still, she hadn't cleared up the confusion over the Warrenders.

By late afternoon, a headache that had been overshadowing Cathy's thoughts had slowly begun to lift and she was able to think clearly. Now she was alone in her consulting room having dismissed her final patient for the day, she considered the facts as she knew them and how she had gradually come to the point she found herself at now.

Initially, she had felt it important to rule out that David Holden had been deliberately targeted. This, Cathy knew, was improbable, as much of the chain of events that had led to his death had been so heavily reliant on chance. Who could have predicted that he would swap guns with Gregory Warrender, after all? Cathy had sought to at least rule out David's wife for completeness. Rosemary Holden had been such an odd woman, and her mother, even more so, being both abrupt and cold, but from their meeting, the one thing that Cathy had decided, was that Rosemary was in deep shock and grieving for the loss of her husband. It seemed clear also, that the young widow was comfortably set up. Her house was plush and the motivation to kill David for ready cash looked highly unlikely.

Of course, there was the other consideration, and Cathy knew the police were now looking into the possibility that Gregory had himself altered the gun, intending to kill David. Cathy had struggled to find a motivation for him doing this, but when she had heard about David's land and estate agency firm showing an interest in the Dewhurst estate, she had seen, at least a loose reason for Gregory to act so decisively. A man so deeply embedded in his farming traditions, with his home and his life rooted there, might quite possibly resort to anything to retain that idyllic existence. But something had rankled, perhaps because it had not been an idyllic existence for Gregory at all. In fact, from what she had heard, the man had been ill-tempered both at home and work a lot of the time. No, it didn't quite fit, and she hoped that the police would draw the same conclusion. Whatever happened, she knew that Gregory, without cause for charge, would be released soon enough.

Cathy crossed to her window and looked out at the already dark sky. Her suspicions had moved on since the initial uncertainties over Gregory's character. Granted, he seemed an unpleasant man, but that was no reason to judge him capable of murder. No, she had transferred her attentions to the more likely theory that Gregory had been the intended victim. It certainly seemed to Cathy more probable that only accident had led to it being David taking the gun from the farmhand at the final moment. She ran through all the people she knew who had reason to wish Gregory dead. What a perplexing list it was. His wife, it seemed, was top of that list, with a motive of both escaping her husband's brutality, and finding solace in her lover. Of course, Kenneth too had the same reasons for wanting Gregory dealt with. How hard it must have been to stand by helplessly watching Fiona's personality crumble. Both Kenneth and Fiona had the opportunity too. Both had been at the shoot that day. Cathy considered the words that Fiona had been overheard whispering. Were they of significance? Had the young woman been urging Kenneth to hurry up and sabotage Gregory's gun while everyone's backs were turned? If she had chosen then to interfere with the gun, might it suggest that the thing had been done on the fly, perhaps without premeditation? But it was still horrific to contemplate. Had the two lovers used the unfortunate accident of Adam Foster's drowning dog to commit their crime? It did seem rather cunning and unlikely when there must surely have been a thousand other opportunities to kill the man had they really wished to do so.

Cathy thought again of her odd visit to the Warrenders' house that day, and how strangely Fiona had behaved. She considered Kenneth and his apparent desire to shield the young woman. In speaking with Rosemary afterwards, Cathy had discovered something else quite new, and her list of suspects had increased consequently. According to Rosemary, for whatever reason, Gregory had been awarded a promotion and a pay increase. Gregory, usually hostile towards the estate manager, had suddenly seemed to change his opinion. The men had been heard laughing together. Why was that?

Cathy thought back to her interview with the estate manager earlier that morning. Certainly, Adam had not given the impression of being on particularly friendly terms with Gregory. Why then, had the farmhand been awarded a raise in pay?

Cathy heard the back-door to the practice slam and a light came on, illuminating Michelle's figure as she crossed the car park, leaving work for the week. Thank goodness it was a Friday. The weekend at least might offer her a chance to reflect on the problem. Cathy watched from her window as the receptionist crossed the street, making her way home to her young family. Cathy had been sitting here for far too long. She must head home herself. She was making little progress worrying over things anyway.

Before logging out of her computer, she checked her emails. The bloody GP supervisor had sent her another message urging her to arrange an appointment for a revalidation interview. What was wrong with the bothersome woman? Cathy had already replied, explaining that James was absent and they would get back in touch as soon as he returned. Of course, what with the Warrender business, Cathy had quite forgotten about completing her paperwork for the dreaded interview. She still had to send out patient and staff questionnaires, which had to be completed as part of it. Cathy felt rather sick at the prospect. Undoubtedly, her attention recently had not been on her work. She hoped that this had gone unnoticed by her colleagues and patients.

This thought concerned her enough to do at least some

preparation for her interview that evening, but her heart certainly wasn't in it. She finally admitted defeat and left a freshly printed stack of staff and patient questionnaires on her desk. These would have to be randomly distributed over the coming week and their responses collated and fed back to her supervisor at the meeting.

That night, it took Cathy a long time to drift off to sleep, and when she did so, it was to fitfully dream of the frightful outcome of her feedback forms. In her nightmare, Mr Duncan had been unable to leave a comment. Cathy had seen herself badgering him for the return of the form, only to find that he had died without her knowledge. Gregory Warrender had, on the other hand, given her excellent feedback. He had written on his questionnaire that Cathy had done him a 'massive favour' in signing his gun licence. When Cathy's supervisor had read this aloud to her, she had tried to defend it, but her mouth had been dry and the words sounded hollow and empty. Finally, Cathy had urged the woman to look at her staff reviews, feeling sure that the practice team would have rated her highly, despite the mix up with her patients. Julie's form was read out first. 'Rude when I came to ask her a question. Dismissive and distracted. Can't be contacted in an emergency,' the girl had scrawled. Cathy had begged the supervisor not to refuse her revalidation. 'My job is everything to me,' she kept saying. 'I'll do anything you want, just name it.' The supervisor had laughed cruelly. 'If I do that, you'll owe me for the rest of your life.'

Cathy had awoken in the early hours gasping. On her lips was the word: 'blackmail.'

Of course, she scolded herself, now fully awake, how could she have been so foolish? Why else might Gregory have been offered a sudden pay rise by Adam Foster? But what did Gregory know about Adam? And was it reason enough for the estate manager to want him dead?

43

'I'm sorry to call on the weekend,' Cathy said to the woman who answered the door.

She looked aloof but nodded and asked her to come in. Cathy stood awkwardly in the great hallway. The last time she had visited, Mr Dewhurst had greeted her and taken her through directly. Now, as she waited, she looked up at the paintings and then to the high ceiling, with its ornate cornice. In the centre, she saw the coat of arms that she had seen also imprinted in gold on the gun cases down at the estate office. She recalled the Latin family motto and its translation: *Invicta veritate*, by invincible truth. That was, after all, why she had come: to find out the truth. It seemed ironic that the person who might hold the key to it had been the one who entrusted her with its solution originally.

That morning, as she had driven up to the big house, she had been surprised to see Gregory's car parked outside the Warrenders' cottage. It seemed likely then, that the police had released him the night before, presumably deciding that what evidence they had was not substantial enough to press charges. Cathy wondered what sort of a reception Gregory had received coming home. Had Kenneth still been there when he returned, and how had Fiona reacted?

Above her, she heard a door open. Turning, she saw Mr Dewhurst slowly descending the stairs.

'Back again, Doctor?' he called, his voice echoing down the stairwell. 'I'm not in any trouble, am I? I thought we had agreed that I should come to you for checkups? I certainly didn't think that my high blood pressure would warrant a house visit on a Saturday.'

Cathy smiled. 'It's not so much a medical visit,' she said.

As he reached the bottom of the stairs he sighed. 'Ah, I see. Well, you'd better come through then, hadn't you?'

Mr Dewhurst led the way into a formal living room. He gestured for her to sit and when she did so, he lowered himself also.

'Well then? I assume it's about the rather delicate matter we discussed before?'

'The fatal shooting, yes. I've just driven past and I see Gregory's car's back. The police haven't pressed charges then, I assume?'

'The detective in charge of the case telephoned yesterday afternoon. No. They seem to have drawn a blank, although they did say that for now, Gregory was not completely cleared from their inquiries, but then, no-one has been from what I can tell. I did tell you that I had my doubts about the local constabulary's ability to get to the bottom of it.'

'Which was why you asked me.'

'Indeed.'

'Well, I have been making a few unofficial explorations into the business,' Cathy said feeling herself blush.

The old man inclined his head. 'What have you got to tell me?'

Cathy grimaced. 'As yet, I'm still unclear, but I did rather hope you'd be able to answer a few questions that had arisen.'

Mr Dewhurst cleared his throat. 'Well, Doctor?'

'More than anything, I'd like to know about Mr Foster, your estate manager,' Cathy said. 'I don't suppose you have had any concerns about him? About his managerial abilities, particularly when dealing with the land,' she paused. 'And possibly, in dealing with your money.'

Mr Dewhurst rubbed his cheek. 'Adam Foster? In many ways, he's been invaluable. It must be said that his employment has allowed me to take a step back, to wind down. He came to us around five years ago, and with good references too. He's a bit of a know-it-all and I understand that he rubs some of the farmhands up the wrong way, but that's inevitable when it comes to dealing with these people.'

'Can you tell me why he promoted Gregory Warrender two weeks ago? His wages were increased dramatically it seems. I assume you know that.'

The old man's cheeks reddened. 'I'll need to speak to Adam. Of course, he has some flexibility in managing the employees. I assumed it was only a very minor increase, and so he felt it unnecessary to bother me.'

Cathy nodded, but she knew that even as he spoke the words, the old man was worried.

'Will you allow me to be completely frank with you, Mr Dewhurst? I feel that I must speak the truth. So many misunderstandings have occurred simply because of the lack of real honesty here.'

He looked steadily at her but didn't contradict.

'Correct me if I'm wrong, but I think you knew that Adam Foster was up to something, am I right? Money has been tight perhaps, and you had begun to look into things yourself possibly. Maybe it appeared that every lead ended back at the estate office. I think you suspected also, that he had something to do with David Holden's death. I couldn't understand why you were so determined to have me look into the thing. If it turned out that your cattleman was guilty, it could hardly impact on you or your reputation. Adam Foster, however, was a different matter. A trusted member of staff. Your own estate manager. I believe that you certainly feared that he had been involved in the death. You were concerned that the embarrassment might sully the name of your family if the police became involved. That's why, I believe, you chose me. A local doctor with a known history of solving puzzles of this kind, but in such a way that it might be easily hushed up. Am I far off the mark?'

Cathy knew that she was not, because the old man's face had paled.

'I'm not accusing you of anything, Mr Dewhurst, but I do think that you know more than you let on. I also believe that Gregory Warrender found out about your estate manager. I assume he walked in and caught Adam fiddling the books in some way. What a gift for the young farmworker, having been spoken down to for so long by Adam. How galling it must have been to devote his life to your farm and the cattle, only to see Adam rewarded for his spineless efforts. I believe that Gregory has been blackmailing Adam Foster in promise for his silence. I doubt it's been going on for long. There seems to have been a dramatic change in their relationship only recently. Perhaps you have been thinking of how to deal with this whole issue for a while now. I must confess that I probably know less about it than you do. I focused on the accident that day rather than your finances.'

Mr Dewhurst looked exhausted. 'You know a good deal,' he said. 'Yes, it's common knowledge that the estate has been struggling. We run the shoots obviously, for additional income, but it's not enough. Adam has only been on my radar these last few months, as it happens. I had noticed that some of the expenditures seemed to be out of kilter. It was difficult to go crashing in without evidence. As I say, he's been with me for five years and in many ways, I'd struggle without him.'

'I can see that you have some painful decisions to make,' Cathy said. 'I can't help with that perhaps, but I do want to talk a little about the man who died, if I may? When I spoke with you before, you mentioned that David Holden had been looking into taking on the land, either to purchase or develop for houses. You were adamant that that wouldn't happen though.'

'I still am,' the old man said. 'Things are desperate but I'd not stoop to selling off fields and ruining my outlook. Having to drive past nasty, little houses to get up my driveway? No thank you.'

'In your own words, you say that it's common knowledge that the estate is in difficulty. I was wondering if you had received any other propositions?'

'You mean the road people, I suppose?'

Cathy nodded. It had taken her a while to remember where she had heard the name before, but it had come to her that morning in the shower. Fiona Warrender worked as an office assistant for Greysons, the road development company. They had been on the news recently, having secured a deal to begin work on a flyover in the area.

'They contacted me, yes,' the old man said. He exhaled. 'Initially, you can imagine my reaction. I told them that they could look elsewhere.'

'But they were presumably quite persuasive?'

The old man sighed. 'I simply agreed to meet with the managing director, Alfie Greyson. I told him that I'd make no promises. He came out to the house and tried to flatter me. He made the proposition out to be a very minor imposition. They'd not wanted much of the land, you see? It was only a single field that they needed. The plan was to straighten the road from Glainkirk and Forkieth. It's well known for accidents being single-track and I believe, there was a huge benefit to the local economy in allowing more traffic through.'

Cathy nodded, recalling the winding country lanes that she had found so troublesome herself. 'So, they didn't suggest cutting right through?'

'Oh goodness, no. I'd have said an outright no to that. It was tempting because it was such a small portion. Barely four or five acres of land, and right on the edge of my estate. The offer they made me was almost too good to refuse.'

'Almost?'

'Well, what with the man's death, I stalled a bit. I told them I needed more time to think. My father taught me that if you had any doubts about a thing, then they were usually well-founded.'

'You thought that the deal was wrong?'

'Just a feeling,' Mr Dewhurst said. 'But I still can't see how this has any bearing on the business with Adam Foster or, for that matter, the fatal shooting. I can promise you, that I will get to the bottom of this business with Adam though. If he has been playing me for a fool, I'll have to let him go I suppose.'

Cathy sighed. 'To be honest, I don't know how it all fits together. I wonder now about Adam, and I suggest that you don't speak to him about this, just for the time being. I'd hate to alert him to my suspicions if he has in some way been involved in the accident.' Cathy shook her head sadly at her muddled thinking. 'No, I think what I must do, is speak to Mr Warrender, now that he seems to be at home. If he's not guilty of the crime, he must surely have his own theory about it. After all, if Gregory was the killer's target, he of all people should know who would wish him dead.'

44

Cathy was disappointed to see that Gregory's car had disappeared when she emerged from her meeting with Mr Dewhurst. Perhaps he had gone to check on his precious cattle. She parked her car at the side of the track, wondering how long she should wait for him to return. She needed to visit someone later, but for the next hour, her day was her own. She hoped Gregory would return soon so that she could ask him outright what he thought of the whole thing. Surely, he must have some idea what had happened that fateful day.

She had parked slightly uphill from the cottage so that if Fiona was to look out, she would not immediately see her car. She didn't want to go knocking on the Warrenders' door unnecessarily, given the rather uncomfortable encounter the previous day. Strange how the tables had turned. At the beginning of all of this, she had been fearful for Fiona's safety, now the girl was on her list of suspects for attempting to kill her husband. Which one of them was the genuine victim?

When it came down to it, only three people could have possibly wanted Gregory dead. His wife, her lover and the object of his blackmail: Adam Foster. Cathy wondered how Gregory might have been feeling all of this time, knowing that he was the one targeted? How had it felt for those first few nights following David's death, to lie with his wife perhaps sleeping in the next room? Had Gregory suspected her?

Cathy recalled again Fiona's panic-stricken words when she had consulted her only the previous week. 'I'm frightened,' the young woman had said. 'Really frightened. What if the police think this wasn't an accident? What if they think Gregory was somehow involved? What if you send me home tonight and I'm sleeping beside a murderer?' Had what the young woman said been a sham? Had Fiona acted hysterically to divert attention from herself? Cathy was sickened at her stupidity if it turned out to be true. But, when all was said and done, who had a better opportunity to kill Gregory than his wife? Why though, had she waited until the day of the shoot? That method was so random and so many things might have gone wrong with the plan, as indeed they seemed to have done.

Cathy sighed. Notably, she was still unclear what the murderer had done to the gun to make it backfire. She remembered what the detective had told her when he had come to the practice asking about Gregory. There had been obvious marks inside the barrel. Cathy knew little of the mechanics of firearms, but perhaps the killer had been inexperienced also. What might one do to make a gun backfire? The obvious thought was to stuff something deep down inside the barrel, hoping that this would lodge and prevent the bullet firing forward and instead cause the rebound explosion in the gun holder's face. What could someone use to do this though? It would have to be something solid enough to prevent a bullet from firing, yet small enough to fit inside. Another bullet perhaps?

Cathy shivered. She had been sitting in the cold car for far too long and her joints ached. She turned on the engine and waited for the heater to kick in. What time was it now? She was becoming restless waiting. Where on earth was Gregory anyway? Cathy looked at the clock. It was nearly one already and she still had another appointment to keep.

'Come on, Gregory,' she moaned.

But after a further ten minutes of waiting, Cathy was cross and frozen through, despite the hot air blasting in her face.

'Damn it,' she cursed and inwardly vowed to return later that day if necessary, to get to the bottom of the problem.

It was a relief to be moving once more and with a purpose. Cathy set off perhaps faster than she should, eager to make the most of what remained of her day. So far, she had achieved little other than confirming her suspicions about Adam Foster being blackmailed. She accelerated onto the road, driving away from the Warrenders' house and towards Glainkirk. As she drove, she looked right and saw through the trees the mansion house which was had been the Dewhurst family home for generations. Continuing for perhaps a mile, she came to a junction in the road and as she waited for a gap in the traffic, she looked again, this time to the open field with what looked like a copse of trees and a river running along the far side. Was this the piece of land that Mr Dewhurst had considered selling to make the road straighter? It was certainly far enough from the main house to have little impact on his outlook.

By the time she reached Glainkirk, Cathy was relieved. She stopped her car outside the grocers and collected a few essentials and then continued on her way, this time, turning towards Forkieth. The hospital car park was crowded as she had expected it might be. She saw also, that the parking charges had increased yet again. Cathy collected her ticket from the machine and the barrier went up. She had no idea what ward he would be on, but she'd find out soon enough.

'I'm looking for a gentleman who was admitted yesterday.

I'm unsure what ward he went to,' she said to the receptionist in the main concourse.

'Hold on a second,' the harassed woman said and finished typing. She then looked up. 'Name?'

Cathy gave it and the woman directed her to ward thirty-four.

'Through to the end, past the sandwich shops, take the first corridor off to the right and ...'

'I've got it,' Cathy said and turned from the desk.

It took her a matter of minutes to find the ward and rather than ask one of the busy nurses fielding questions from an irate family, she looked at the whiteboard above the nurses' station and saw the name. Mr Duncan had been allotted bay two, bed three.

He didn't notice her at first, even when she drew up a chair beside his bed, but when he did, his face was pitifully grateful.

'How are you?' she asked him. 'I'm glad to see you sitting up and looking brighter.'

He shook his head. 'What are you doing coming in to see me on a weekend? I take it you were in seeing someone else?'

'Not at all,' she said fiercely and then smiled. 'What the verdict then?'

'Food's not great,' he said and smiled. 'Feel a bit of a fraud. Heartburn, that's all it was, heartburn! And I called an ambulance for that.'

'You were frightened. Calling nine-nine-nine was exactly the right thing to do in the circumstances. I'm sorry. I feel I've rather let you down recently. If I had been more attentive, made myself more available ...'

The old man shook his head and touched her hand with his. His skin was cold. 'You're not to blame. You have other people to care for besides me.'

'Have they mentioned when you might get home? I assume,

not over the weekend? We'll perhaps need to organise a few services to come in and help a little, only until you're feeling a bit more settled. I've been to the shops already and picked up a few things just in case.'

His eyes were tear-filled. 'Not told me yet. I've not minded being here so much. They're nice, the nurses. It's nice to have company. You shouldn't have gone to that bother, you know?'

Cathy sat with him for an hour and listened, really listened, with her focus entirely on the man. He spoke to her about his beloved wife and recounted stories of bygone days, laughing that he'd not thought about them in a long while. When Cathy got up to leave, she felt somehow lighter. In the last hour, she too had laughed a good deal and perhaps this freeing of emotion had done her as much good as her patient.

Returning to her car, she sighed. Well, she'd made little headway with the Warrenders, but she had at least made things right with Mr Duncan.

The parking ticket had slid down the side of her purse. Cathy fumbled trying to get the thing out while behind her, she was aware of the growing queue. Three pounds, the machine told her when she slid the ticket into the slot. Three pounds. It was outrageous. Cathy knocked on the side of her purse, counting out the change. One pound fifty. Was that a fifty pence piece?

And then it hit her. She almost lost balance with the realisation and found herself staring unseeingly at the man behind her in the queue.

'Are you going to pay then?' he asked.

Cathy shook her head and smiled. 'No,' she said and began laughing. 'Oh my God! How can I have been so stupid? And it was there under the stairs the whole time!'

The man tutted and shook his head. 'Loony,' he mumbled and pushed past her.

45

With shaking hands, Cathy made a call from her mobile. At first, she thought that the woman wouldn't allow her to speak to him, but eventually, she did and he confirmed what she had suspected. 'Please don't mention this conversation to anyone,' she begged. 'Not until I'm sure.' Hanging up, she sighed. Motive enough certainly, but which one of them had done it?

She was unaware of driving home from the hospital at all. But once there, Cathy paced up and down in her kitchen. 'Think,' she told herself. 'Think.' The harder she tried to force it though, the worse it became. By late afternoon, and with the evening fast drawing in, her head throbbed with the effort. Knowing that she was making little progress, she gave it up and made herself watch the television. Nothing much was on and she found her mind beginning to wander once again. Impulsively, she snatched up her mobile.

'Are you alright to talk?'

'Yes, always for you.'

Cathy sighed. 'Sorry, I forgot even what shifts you were on this week. My head's a mess.'

'Revalidation worries again?' Suzalinna asked and then Cathy heard her friend cupping her hand over the phone. 'Not there, Saj. I told you in the kitchen. Sorry, Darling,' she said. 'Saj is unable to take even the simplest of instructions.'

Cathy laughed. 'Oh, Suz. You've no idea how lucky you are to have that man.' She sighed again. 'Suz, I'm in a bit of a mess. My head's scrambled.'

'What do you mean? You're not unwell again? You've been taking your medication, haven't you?'

Cathy smiled. 'Not that. No, it's not that at all. I feel I've let a few people down recently, not least of all, a number of patients. James is coming back next week. I had wanted the practice to be in good order. I think I've fallen rather short.'

'Well, you said yourself, locums are tricky. We've got a hellish registrar at the moment covering for Brodie. Awful, he is. Swans in and out, leaves the juniors alone in resus. God help us if he's ever promoted to consultant. He won't be employed in my department anyway. No darling, locums are always hopeless. They never do the job as a regular doctor might and yet, they get paid almost twice as much. Listen, how can you expect things to be as good as if both you and James were there? I know you had a point to prove, but that pressure was of your own making. I'll bet James would be horrified if he knew how uptight you've been in his absence. What about the other business? Has someone been charged, do you know? I had heard a rumour ...'

Cathy groaned. 'The police released their main suspect, but I had my doubts about it being him from the very start.'

'What about the young girl? The parasuicide? I asked Frances and she said she'd been discharged from the short stay ward the following morning. Paracetamol levels and so on were all OK. The only thing they found was mild hypoxia when she first came in. I assume it just booze then? What do you think?'

'Maybe,' Cathy said. 'She's been on my mind a good deal. I

visited her at home after her hospital stay. Strange. I do wonder if she has some kind of psychotic illness brewing. Nothing concrete, but she's quite paranoid at times. It's odd because when she came to the surgery to see me the first time, she didn't give that impression at all. She seemed like a normal girl. Frightened perhaps of her husband, but not delusional.'

'Well darling, I'm glad James is back on Monday to help. It sounds as if you've been stressing out.'

Cathy rubbed her forehead. 'I've had a splitting headache,' she admitted.

'Go to bed and rest,' her friend advised. 'Will we catch up next week, do you think? I'll come to you and I'll even help you cobble together some nonsense for your revalidation paperwork if you like. We'll have a brainstorming session like when we were students, do you remember?'

Cathy laughed. 'Thanks,' she said. 'I'd be lost without you.'

'Oh, before you go, Cath. I suppose the girl told you when you visited her that she was pregnant, did she?'

Cathy froze. 'What?'

'Yes, well that was your hunch wasn't it? Frances persuaded her to have her urine checked and right enough, she was. Hopefully, her boozy binge won't have impacted the foetus. Must have decided against taking those morning-after-pills that you found. Probably flushed them down the loo.'

Cathy unexpectedly felt completely spent. When she hung up the phone, she stood motionless for some time. So, Fiona had been pregnant all along. Suddenly, more than anything, all Cathy wanted to do was to crawl into bed. Her mind had been so active all day, and having spoken with her friend, it was as if a switch had been flicked. She must eat something though if she hoped to shift her headache.

She filled the kettle and slotted a couple of slices of bread into the toaster. The kettle began to hum and the smell of the toast made her spirits lift. She buttered the toast and then decided that jam too would be the right thing. When she had finished, she took a mug of tea and a hot water bottle that she had had the foresight to fill also, and climbed the stairs.

In the bathroom, she splashed her face with water. With blinking eyes, she looked at her blotchy reflection. What was it that she was missing? Something stirred in Cathy's memory. She recalled Fiona's face when she had gone to the house the other day. The girl had been insensible with drink. Her cheeks had been blotchy-red also. What had Suzalinna said on the phone just now? They had checked the girl's oxygen saturations and she had been mildly hypoxic on admission to accident and emergency. Cathy dropped the towel she had been holding to dry her face. Oh God, but it all fitted with the symptoms then. How could she have been so utterly stupid? Cathy looked about herself. She had to do something. If it was so, then she couldn't leave it a moment longer.

With her heart hammering in her throat, she ran downstairs. Oh God, what if she was too late? How could she have been so slow to spot the signs? But who should she call? She had no-one's numbers as they were all on the computer at the practice. The only person close enough to intervene was Mr Dewhurst himself. She didn't like to call the old man at such an hour. If she had had Adam Foster's number, she might have called him. But she had no choice. Cathy grabbed her car keys from the hall table and as she forced her feet into her trainers, she waited for the call to be answered.

The drive took forever, the roads at night seeming more convoluted and dangerous than even during the day. The temperature had dropped considerably too, and several times, the car tyres slid. But Cathy could not slow down and instead, she pressed on, her headlights catching the hedgerows as she went. At one point, she saw the flapping of wings and a roosting pheasant swung out and across her path. This time, Cathy did not need to swerve though, and the bird lifted up and above the car, screaming an indignant cry. 'Come on, come on,' she repeated under her breath, willing the miles to disappear and the turn off to loom out from the dark. If she was too late, she might never forgive herself.

When she finally turned onto the road leading to the estate, she saw several lights ahead of her. It seemed then, that her telephone call had had the desired effect. Pulling off the track and parking her car, she was aware of another car's headlights snaking behind her on the road that led to the estate. Cathy didn't wait to see who followed, but instead, marched up the path to the house. Her heart was beating fast and her hands shook. Mr Dewhurst and Kenneth were already there standing on the front step.

'No answer,' Mr Dewhurst said.

'Are they both inside?' Cathy asked and turned to see Kenneth's serious countenance. 'Oh, Christ. We have to get in,' she said.

She looked and unfortunately, it appeared that Adam Foster had been diligent and had organised for the front door to be entirely replaced.

'We've tried it already,' Kenneth said. 'It won't budge this time. Adam got a company out and they made too good a job of it. We've been calling and throwing stones up, but they've not woken.'

'Look,' Mr Dewhurst said. 'If this is as grave an emergency as you suggest, then I do think we should just break a window.'

Cathy nodded.

They were joined then by Adam Foster, who must have been the person following Cathy along the Glainkirk Road.

'Ah Adam,' Mr Dewhurst said. 'Did you bring a spare key?

We can't get the door in, and we were going to have to smash a window.'

Adam didn't speak, but elbowed past them and fumbled with the lock. Then, the door was open and they all tumbled inside. There was a good deal of shouting and Cathy called for Kenneth and Adam to get all the doors and windows open as fast as they could. But Kenneth was ahead of her, racing up the stairs to the Warrenders' bedroom.

'Fiona!' he screamed. 'Fiona wake up!'

Cathy was close behind him. Kenneth flung open the door that she knew led to the main bedroom. She heard him shouting and then a woman groan. Cathy instead turned to the other door and opening this, flicked on the light. In bed, lay Gregory Warrender. His face was red and mottled. Cathy rushed to the window and opened it. Already her head was swimming.

'Get her outside if you can,' she called through to the other room, hearing Kenneth now talking firmly.

With the windows open, the house was quite bitterly cold. She didn't have to wait long for Gregory to wake. In the hallway, she could hear the others talking. It seemed that, with Adam's assistance, they were getting Fiona safely down the stairs.

'Gregory!' Cathy said. 'Wake up, Gregory.'

The breeze from the open window suddenly gusted and the curtain flapped. Gregory stirred and then his eyelids flickered.

'What's going on?' he mumbled and Cathy herself, began to breath more easily.

It didn't take long for him to come around. Adam popped his head around the door.

'Make sure the boiler's off, Adam. I assume that's what it was. Carbon monoxide poisoning. I should have realised sooner. Fiona had all the symptoms. Headache, red face, agitation, and it was always when she'd been in the house for some time.'

Adam nodded and disappeared once again.

Gregory now sat up in bed. Cathy shivered and he too must have felt the cold because he instinctively drew the covers up further.

'Sorry,' she said, 'the window stays open for now. When you feel a little more like yourself Mr Warrender, perhaps we can have a little talk. I think you know as well as I do, that you've been a very lucky man. To escape death once is fortunate, but twice, really is lucky.'

46

Cathy closed the bedroom door. She had checked that an ambulance had been called, more out of precaution than anything, given that both Mr and Mrs Warrender were now quite lucid. In fact, Fiona was speaking quite animatedly downstairs, seemingly enjoying the attention the events of that night had afforded her. When Cathy had last looked, Kenneth had been hunting around for a blanket to wrap around Fiona's knees and Adam and Mr Dewhurst were talking quietly about how could it have been that they had allowed the boiler to be in such a state that it had nearly caused a fatality in one of their rented cottages. Someone should have been checking, Mr Dewhurst had been saying severely. Cathy left them to it and returned to Gregory.

'The ambulance will be here soon,' she said. 'I wanted a word first though. So much has happened this past week, since the shooting.'

Gregory nodded.

'I'm afraid that you were chief suspect for a good while,' Cathy laughed. 'Not only with the police, but with me also. Mr Dewhurst asked me to look into the business, you see?'

'It wasn't me at all. I know they all say it was. I hardly knew the man, for God's sake. I said it a thousand times to the police. They seemed to think that it had something to do with his company wanting to build houses on the farmland. Said that I must really love my job and see it as more of a vocation than anything.'

'Well, that bit was true, I suppose,' Cathy said. 'But no, I soon realised that the target had not been David Holden. After all, the gun had only ended up in his hands by chance. That, of course, only left one person as the intended victim. You. It was planned quite deliberately. In cold blood. Not an impulsive decision at all, but a carefully planned one.'

'I suppose it was when Adam's dog fell in the river that they did it?' Gregory asked. 'I was in the bushes and someone was behind me. I'm sure it was Kenneth who pushed me in. He's the only person.'

'He had scratches on his knuckles, presumably as he scrambled towards the river,' Cathy said.

'Oh, you saw that too? Yes, I noticed. It only occurred to me when I was at the police station. There was so much commotion that day. I wracked my brains while I was sitting in that cell, trying to think whose face I didn't see. Who could have been at my car boot, meddling with the gun?'

'Admittedly, if it was Kenneth in the bushes with you and he pushed you into the river, that was a dreadful thing to do.'

'I might well have been swept away. The river was high.'

'But not quite attempted murder, was it? And if it was Kenneth in the bushes with you, he could hardly be rooting around in your car boot, could he? Anyway, I'm not so sure it was then, that they did it.'

Gregory nodded. 'I suppose you know what they used?'

Cathy laughed. 'It took me a while to work it out. It had to be something small enough to fit in the barrel and lodge, but hard enough to stop the bullet from forcing forwards. A coin, of course. I was very slow with that.'

'I found it on the ground after he was taken away by the ambulance. Lying at my feet in amongst the grass.'

'But it wasn't just any coin, was it?'

Gregory's eyes widened. 'How on earth can you possibly know?'

Cathy laughed. 'I'm afraid I was desperately looking to clear your name. When Fiona was taken unwell, I'll admit, I did have a look around the house. It was partly to see if she had swallowed anything she shouldn't, but also to search for clues.' Cathy crossed the room to the dressing table. 'In here,' she said. 'I saw the metal-detector under the stairs too.'

Gregory nodded and signalled for her to open the drawer. 'I suppose it was daft really to think that I could keep it a secret. I was a bit of a fool and boasted to David about it when he came for dinner the night before anyway. I even showed the coins to him. I was drunk and stupid. I'd have had to tell Mr Dewhurst of course, but the thought, you see, of sitting on all that treasure ...'

'Yes, I can imagine it was a thrill. You found this in one of the estate fields?' she asked, holding up a coin from the box.

'Potter's field. It's where we were shooting when the accident happened. I thought someone might have seen me the last time I had been out metal-detecting. Something flashed. I thought it was a light in the trees and then, I wondered if it was binoculars trained on me. I thought that gamekeeper Kenneth had been the one ...'

Cathy sighed. 'He's given you a headache for a while now, I believe?'

'Fiona said they were just friends, but I knew something was going on. I'm not stupid. The thought that I knew about the Roman treasure trove gave me at least some joy. It was childish really, but I liked knowing that Fiona didn't know, if you see what I mean?'

'And you knew other things too ...'

'My God! You do dig around, don't you? I doubt Adam would have told you though. Yes, I found out about him fiddling the books. I'm not proud of myself, but I did feel that, after years of working for the estate, I deserved some compensation.'

'You blackmailed him.'

'You could put it like that. Mr Dewhurst was a fool to trust him in the first place.'

'Oh, I wouldn't call Mr Dewhurst a fool at all,' Cathy said, shaking her head. 'He's more astute than you'd think.' And to Gregory's puzzled expression, she continued. 'He has suffered some financial trouble recently. I presume the police told you that David's company planned to make Mr Dewhurst an offer? They wanted to buy up his land and build houses on it.'

Gregory snorted. 'He'd not have done that. Not ever.'

'No, perhaps not. But he was made another offer also.'

Gregory looked surprised.

'An offer by a different company. This was a far more substantial offer, but not only that. It would only involve buying a very small portion of the land. A corner, right on the edge. Barely four acres maximum. In fact, it was so tempting, given that the land was peripheral and of little necessity to the estate, that Mr Dewhurst was seriously considering it.'

'Why would anyone want four acres? What use would that be?'

'Greysons ...'

Gregory looked astonished. 'What? Fiona's company? The road people?'

Cathy nodded. 'That's right. It seems that there have been plans for a while now, to straighten out the road between Glainkirk and Forkieth. The narrow, winding country lanes don't offer access to larger vehicles. I know, from bitter experience, how simple it is to misjudge a bend.' Cathy smiled, but Gregory looked ashen. 'The deal, if it took place, would have been of immense benefit to Greysons. I suspect that they were desperate to ensure that it went through.'

'You can't mean? But why me? Why would anyone try to kill me? What had I to stop them from going ahead? I'm only a cattleman.'

'Sadly, you were a big problem, Gregory, because of exactly what we've just spoken of: the Roman artefacts. Had they been realised, there would be no way a road could ever go through that field. Months, and months, if not years, of excavations, would need to take place to ensure that all the relics were uncovered. Even then, with the deal already precarious given Mr Dewhurst's reluctance to sell, the moment might pass. The old man could easily get cold feet and change his mind. Or his fortunes, following the Roman treasure discovery, might alter to such a degree that there would be no incentive for him to sell up at all.'

Gregory looked horrified. 'Oh God,' he whispered. 'Then I was right all along. I thought it was because of her and Kenneth, but it was because of Greysons all the time. That bloody company. That bloody job. I knew as soon as she took it, it meant the end for us.'

Cathy sighed, but before they could speak further, she heard a piercing wail. For a moment, Cathy thought it was the siren of an approaching ambulance, but she then realised that it came from the stairs. Fiona Warrender had overheard all that they had said.

'Can I see her?' Cathy asked.

The previous hour seemed to have passed in a blur. The ambulances had come and both Mr and Mrs Warrender had been stretchered into them. The police had been present also, which was probably just as well given the circumstances.

When she had finished talking to the detective in charge of the case, Cathy had driven, not home, but into Glainkirk, following the path that the ambulances would have taken minutes before as they carried Fiona and Gregory to hospital. Cathy didn't follow them to accident and emergency, but instead turned off the main road and up a side street.

The house was in darkness save for one upstairs light and she wondered if she was wrong to have come. By now, it was almost midnight and no-one would appreciate a call at this time.

The door opened.

'You're too late,' the woman said.

'You can't mean?' Cathy began. 'When?'

'I just found her.'

Rosemary Holden's mother turned and Cathy followed her inside.

The plush, carpeted stairs creaked as the two women ascended them in silence.

'She's in there. It's like she's sleeping.'

Cathy pushed the door.

The room looked immaculate. Everything was in perfect order and even the bedcovers that lay across her were straight and unruffled. Cathy crossed the room and gazed down at the woman's face. Her eyes were closed and the lids were almost a translucent mauve. There was no sign of distress whatsoever. Cathy slid her hand under Rosemary's hair and felt for a pulse, but the temperature of the woman's skin already told her that she had been dead for some hours. Cathy stepped back and glanced around the room.

'In the bathroom,' the elderly woman told her, and she crossed to the other door.

By the sink, in perfect alignment, were three empty packets of sleeping tablets and one of a morphine-based painkiller. Cathy turned in confusion

'They were David's,' the woman explained. 'He had a bad back a few months ago and must have kept hold of them. I didn't realise she was planning it, but perhaps it's just as well.'

Cathy nodded. 'You know why?'

'She told me, yes. I would have come to stay with her anyway after David's death, but she told me outright that she had done it. Ambitious like her father,' the old woman said, shaking her head. 'He'll be devastated, of course. I've not told him yet. Perhaps, I won't tell him the full story now. Why spoil it for him; the impression of his daughter? Let him think that she ended it because she couldn't bear life without David.'

'That's true to a point,' Cathy said and the other woman grimaced.

'It was never like that, and I think you know it. Being married to David can't have been easy. I never got on with him particularly. He did see himself as rather superior to Rosemary. Ridiculous really,' she said and smiled wanly. 'Rosemary had more business sense in her little finger than that foolish, little estate agent ever had. He had plans and great ideas. Out of loyalty, she followed him. She suppressed her ambitions and allowed him to believe that he was the greater intellect. Ridiculous, as I say.' The old woman snorted. 'When she took on the position at Greysons, I think that the managing director saw almost instantly what he was dealing with. She had a drive and accuracy like few other personal assistants. Very quickly, she became heavily involved in many of the decisions. She was so devoted to the company. They could trust her judgment implicitly. David, of course, knew nothing. He couldn't see what was right in front of him, silly man. He was still under the illusion that he was going to seal some farcical deal to propel them out of this small town and somewhere truly great, but it was Rosemary, you see? She was the one.'

'Did the people at Greysons realise what she planned?'

'What? That she intended to kill to push the company's plans through? Oh, I doubt that very much.'

Cathy shook her head. 'It's so sad. To accidentally murder her husband and then regret it.'

The older woman looked confused. 'But I thought you understood,' she said. 'It wasn't accidental at all. It was intentional. Rosemary never allowed anything to run to chance.'

'Are you saying that she intended to kill David? I thought it was Gregory Warrender; the man whose gun David borrowed.'

'Nonsense. That was part of the scheme. It was her idea; to distract attention from herself. Kill two birds with one stone. Let him take the rap for it. She could have killed David at any moment she wanted. If I'd have known about it before, I might have encouraged her.'

Cathy must have looked horrified.

'Well, perhaps not,' the old woman admitted. 'I might well have told her to find another way. The marriage was unhappy though. It had been for some time. I think that she had begun to wonder if this was all her life might amount to.' The old woman gestured around the room. 'No, of course, she planned to kill David. She had to get him out of the way with his silly plan about houses. Mr Dewhurst had become more receptive to the company's approaches, so David had told her. Rosemary knew that was a lie, but she also knew that the more David muddled around, the less likely Greysons would be in managing to negotiate. It's a delicate business and people don't want to be hounded. This Mr Dewhurst sounded like he was old-school. Not the type to stand for that sort of thing. In fudging his own company's chances with the land, David would also risk losing the deal for Greysons. Rosemary couldn't allow that. She said herself it had become a bit of an obsession.'

'I still don't understand how though,' Cathy said. 'I know when she sabotaged the gun, but how could she have known that Gregory would hand it to David?'

The old woman laughed. 'She told me she did it the night before the shoot. Hoped that everyone would assume it was done during the day at some point, although I believe things got muddled when a dog fell in the water. She already knew where the gun was kept, you see? She'd seen it that evening apparently, when Gregory's wife had asked her to get more beer from under the stairs. Left the key to the gun case on the kitchen table, so she said. It was all too easy. Rosemary was good with things like that. Efficient and resourceful. She knew long before about Gregory's metal-detecting nonsense. Fiona had inadvertently told her about it going into work one morning and the weekend before Rosemary had driven out to the estate to take a look at what he was up to. Caught him in the very field Greysons needed. She thought he'd spotted her too. Must have seen a glint on the binoculars. After that, she was quite determined, even more so, when Gregory was drunkenly boasting to David about finding treasure.'

'How could she know though that Gregory wouldn't shoot the gun first?'

'She didn't. She hoped that the shoot would run as it always did. He apparently, didn't normally take part, but always carried his gun. Fiona had told her that. When it came to lunchtime and the two women brought their picnic, Rosemary was rewarded to find that she had been right. Men like Gregory are creatures of habit.'

'But I still can't see how she would know that David would use Gregory's gun.'

'Psychology,' the old woman said. 'Rosemary was so astute. Always was. She spoke to David on the shoot at lunchtime. A group of them were talking. She made a joke out of his shooting abilities and nodded to Gregory. Said he had a better gun. The rest was inevitable. She knew that David wouldn't be able to resist a shot.' She smiled at the irony of what she had said. 'Well, she was right.'

'But when I came to visit her, she seemed so ...'

'Oh yes. I think she knew almost immediately that her plan had been a wretched mistake. She tried to live with it. She confessed the lot to me in the hope that it might ease things.' The old woman looked down at her daughter. 'So beautiful, but so troubled,' the old woman whispered. 'I hope she found the peace she was looking for.'

'Well then darling, what a palaver it's been!'

Cathy grinned at her friend. 'As you say.'

'So, what about the Warrenders? I assume the police recognise that Gregory's not their man?'

'She left a note,' Cathy explained. 'It seems that everything was taken care of. Very like her, according to her poor mother.'

Suzalinna grimaced. 'Horrible for you. Did you suspect her then?'

'I found her a bit odd when I first met her. Initially, I wondered about it being her. The wife is usually the most obvious suspect after all, but she had no motive that I could think of, and when I visited, she seemed utterly distraught. I discounted her from the off and focused on who wanted Gregory dead.'

'And you found a fair few?'

Cathy laughed. 'Well, his wife, obviously, and the gamekeeper.'

'They were having an affair, weren't they?'

Cathy shook her head. 'I assumed that too, but no, it really was innocent. They were just friends. Kenneth, I think, was fiercely protective of her. The way Fiona carried on, he thought the same as me; that her husband was beating her, although I don't think she ever said that. Fiona was all over the place as it was.'

'The carbon monoxide poisoning? I assume the estate manager will be in trouble for not seeing to the maintenance?'

'He's gone. Mr Dewhurst was reluctant to fire him despite the fraud, funnily enough. I think Adam Foster was as close as the old man had ever come to having a son. After Mr Dewhurst's wife died, I think he relied on Adam a good deal. He got a good reference in the end,' Cathy said. 'Not that he really deserved it, but he was efficient and I'm sure he'll get another job all too easily.'

'And the estate?'

'Safe and looking financially more hopeful. The field will be excavated and depending on what they find, Mr Dewhurst will make a decision. If they find Roman artefacts, he'll be delighted, of course. If not, he may still sell to Greysons.'

'And the Warrenders plan to stay on, even in the same house?'

'I believe so,' Cathy said.

'But the boiler will obviously get a full service first though?'

Cathy grinned at her friend. 'Well, obviously.'

'I'm annoyed I didn't think of the gas leak,' Suzalinna continued. 'When she was hypoxic, it should have made me think.'

'It had been going on for a while, remember? The boiler was slowly leaking. Not enough to seriously harm them, but Fiona, in particular, seems to have been susceptible to the fumes. She was paranoid and she had headaches all the time. At one point, she thought that Gregory was trying to poison her.'

'But he was the good guy all along.'

Cathy laughed. 'If you like. I never took to him, but he'll have to buck up his ideas now he's going to become a father.'

'Fiona's had no ill-effects from the alcohol or the gas then?'

'Thankfully none, but we'll have to wait and see. I'll see her more regularly throughout the pregnancy along with obstetrics, just to be on the safe side. It seems that, although things were turbulent in the marriage, there was still some love there.'

Suzalinna snorted. 'Enough to make a child anyway.'

'I think she must have panicked when she thought she was pregnant. It was after she and Gregory had had a blazing row. She bought the morning-after-pill in a rage and only realised when she had it, that it was beyond the seventy-two-hour window of taking it. Now, they're both delighted that she didn't take it. Perhaps a child will cement the marriage. I certainly hope so. Poor Fiona was distraught when she overheard Gregory saying that he believed she was the killer. I really think they love one another.' Cathy smiled.

'Right, come on then.' Suzalinna said, lifting the first folder to her right. 'Enough chat. You've been delaying for ages. Let's crack on with the real reason I'm here. Talk me through the duties of a doctor as set out by the General Medical Council.'

'Are you for real?'

Suzalinna raised her eyebrows.

'Oh, for God's sake, Suz.'

Suzalinna was studying the papers in front of her and didn't look up.

Cathy groaned. 'Well, obviously I have a duty to keep up to date with medical advances, as I've demonstrated with all of my course attendances listed there.' Cathy pointed to the form. 'You know this is ridiculous, right?'

Her friend scowled, refusing to drop the role of revalidation assessor.

Cathy sighed. 'Bloody hell, fine. I must be truthful and communicate effectively with my patients ...'

'I see you have patient questionnaires here,' Suzalinna said, still acting the part. She read aloud: "Dr Moreland is sometimes abrupt. She is clearly a busy woman."

'Oh, give me a break,' Cathy begged.

Suzalinna raised a hand to silence her. She continued reading. "But," she read, "despite her hectic schedule, she always finds time, going way above and beyond the call of duty."

Cathy rolled her eyes and blushed.

"Dr Moreland listens to me when I feel like no-one else will." Suzalinna looked up. 'It's not just one. I could go on.' She leafed through the papers. 'You offer more than the average doctor's level of care. Anyone can see that this is your vocation.'

Cathy sighed. 'I hope the assessor agrees next week when James comes back to work.'

Suzalinna smiled wickedly. 'Well darling, if all else fails, you're making a bit of a name for yourself what with all this murder solving. Soon the police will come straight to your door when someone dies. If the medical career goes to pot, you've always got criminal investigation to fall back on!'

Suzalinna then quickly ducked, as a paper folder was hurled towards her.

THANK YOU!

I do hope that you have enjoyed reading Shooting Pains, the third book in the Dr Cathy Moreland Mystery series. If you'd like to hear about future releases and offers, please visit my website http://mairichong.com and sign up to my mailing list. I'd love to have you with me. I'm also often active on Facebook (Mairi Chong Author) and twitter @mairichong. Do pop by and say hello!

Finally, if you have enjoyed the book, please consider recommending it to a friend or writing a review on the site purchased, Goodreads, or Bookbub. It would mean the world to me.

Check out other titles in the Dr Cathy Moreland Mystery Series

ACKNOWLEDGMENTS

Firstly, thank you to John Ferguson. Although we never met, I'd like to imagine you looking down on us now, chuckling about how your beloved wife, Carol ended up advising on guns and pheasants! Dearest Carol, thank you and I love you. To my editor Amanda, a massive thanks. You have been such a great help this year. Many thanks to my parents for their support and encouragement. You are the first to offer to help, yet often the last to get credit for doing so. Please know that I love and appreciate you. As always, thank you to my darling husband, without whom I would be hopelessly lost, and my son, who sat alongside me as I wrote this book, offering helpful (and amusing) plot suggestions!

Finally, thank you to all of the people who told me that they enjoyed *Murder and Malpractice* and *Deadly Diagnosis* enough to want more. Your continued support is so genuinely appreciated. I can't wait to share the next book in the series with you very soon!

Printed in Great Britain
by Amazon

51415949R00154